C000077024

EMERGENCY
PRACTICE

TRIAGE IN
EMERGENCY
PRACTICE

GAIL HANDYSIDES, RN, MSN, CEN, MA(c)
Instructor, School of Nursing
San Diego State University
San Diego, California

with contributions from

RUSSELL HANSCOM, RN, MHA
Internal Consultant
Clinical Planning and Improvement
Group Health Cooperative of Puget Sound
Seattle, Washington

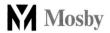 Mosby

St. Louis   Baltimore   Boston
Carlsbad   Chicago   Naples   New York   Philadelphia   Portland
London   Madrid   Mexico City   Singapore   Sydney   Tokyo   Toronto   Wiesbaden

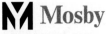

Mosby
Dedicated to Publishing Excellence

A Times Mirror
Company

Publisher: Nancy Coon
Editor: Robin Carter
Editorial Assistant: Kerri Rabbitt
Project Manager: Patricia Tannian

Senior Production Editor: Ann E. Rogers
Senior Design Manager: Gail M. Hudson
Cover Design: Teresa Breckwoldt
Manufacturing Manager: Betty Richmond

Printed in the United States of America
Composition by Wm. C. Brown Group
Printing/binding by R.R. Donnelley and Sons Company

Mosby–Year Book, Inc.
11830 Westline Industrial Drive, St. Louis, Missouri 63146

Library of Congress Cataloging in Publication Data

Handysides, Gail.
    Triage in emergency practice / Gail Handysides, with contributions from Russell Hanscom.
        p. cm.
    Includes bibliographical references and index.
    ISBN 0-8016-7892-7 (spiral)
    1. Triage (medicine) 2. Emergency nursing. I. Hanscom, Russell. II. Title.
    [DNLM: 1. Emergencies—nursing—handbooks. 2. Triage—handbooks. WY 49 H236t 1996]
RC86.7.H366 1996
616.02′5—dc20
DNLM/DLC
for Library of Congress   95–10713
                                                                          CIP

95 96 97 98 99 / 9 8 7 6 5 4 3 2 1

This book is dedicated to my mother

Ouida Sprague Hanscom

who first taught me
that listening is an act of love

and to

Lillian Moore

who first showed me
that nursing and nurturing are truly synonymous

Consultants

CYNTHIA ABEL, RN, MSN, CEN

Assistant Professor in Clinical Nursing
The University of Texas
Houston Health Science Center
Houston, Texas

LINDA GREENBERG, RN, MS, CEN
Director of Emergency-Trauma Services
Sacred Heart Medical Center
Spokane, Washington

JUDY KAYE, ARNP, MSN, CCRN, CS
Critical Care-Neuroscience Clinical Nurse Specialist
University Hospital
Augusta, Georgia

PATRICIA J. KELLY, MS, RN, CEN
Instructor
Harbor Hospital School of Nursing
Baltimore, Maryland

PAMELA STINSON KIDD, RN, PhD, CEN
Assistant Professor, College of Nursing
University of Kentucky
Lexington, Kentucky

LARRY PURNELL, PhD, RN
Associate Professor, College of Nursing
University of Delaware
Newark, Delaware

ANNE RUSSEL, MSN, CCRN
Trauma Clinical Associate
Miami Valley Hospital
Dayton, Ohio

PATRICIA J. STURT, RN, MSN, CEN
Staff Development Specialist
Emergency Department
University of Kentucky
Lexington, Kentucky

JUNE M. THOMPSON, RN, DrPH, CEN
Emergency Medicine
Children's Hospital
Columbus, Ohio

KATHLEEN WALSH, RN, MS, CEN
Clinical Nurse Specialist
Emergency Room
New England Medical Center
Boston, Massachusetts

JEAN WILL, RN, MSN, CEN, EMTP
Vice Chair
Department of Primary Care Education and Community Service
Medical College of Pennsylvania and Hahnemann University
Philadelphia, Pennsylvania

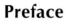

Preface

Many ingredients are necessary for an effective triage system: adequate space, supplies, and communication systems, and access to an area where care is provided. The most essential component of excellent triage care is the professional who provides the care. This person must have a strong knowledge background in assessment, disease processes, public health, and community resources. The professional with experience will have an added benefit of having intuitive abilities in judging the degree of severity a patient's illness or injury represents and the degree of risk to the patient associated with waiting for care. Time-management skills, the ability to cope well with stress, and the maturity to recognize when collaboration with a physician or member of management is indicated are essential for a triage nurse. A compassionate nature and the ability to consider patient comfort at all times are crucial for obtaining complete information and for establishing a trusting relationship with the patient. The trust the triage nurse establishes with a patient will facilitate the patient's receptiveness to care and education once in a treatment area. When triage is performed in an expert and kind manner, excellent public relations for the health care facility is an added benefit.

Triage guidelines provided in this book are intended to serve as organized recommendations for obtaining essential history information relevant to the patient's chief complaint, as well as indicating critical objective assessment data that can practically be obtained in triage. Critical findings are listed in each chapter, and although they may not be all inclusive for every health problem known to emergency care, they represent common indicators that a patient requires medical attention without delay. Specific considerations relevant to geriatric and pediatric populations are integrated throughout the text.

Operationalizing any skill, whether it is in the computer industry, linguistics, medicine, or nursing, should be done only with the intent of providing guidelines. A skill that is over-operationalized does not encourage practitioner freedom to interpret data using professional knowledge and experience. If an individual assigned to triage requires detailed algorithms to make judgments regarding patient acuity, that person has no business performing triage. If the triage professional is a registered nurse who is educated in assessment and triage policies and procedures and has access to resources for information, liability risks for the health care facility will be minimal and patients will receive appropriate triage designations and care.

Gail Handyside

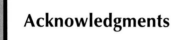

Acknowledgments

I would like to acknowledge my family for their understanding and patience: my husband Roger, who couldn't get to sleep when I was writing halfway into the night, and my children Jeremy, Sonja, and Julie, who continued to love me even when I wasn't always there to provide the support they needed. Special thanks to the Daughters of Charity and the staff of St. Vincent's residential program for the developmentally disabled who nurture Sonja and without whose help this book could not have been conceived or realized.

I want to thank my colleagues at Palomar Medical Center and San Diego State University for all they have taught me and the Palomar-Pomerado Hospital District for allowing me to photograph patients in their facilities. My photographer Rudy Vaca and all the patients whom he photographed were so helpful and kind. Thanks to Helme Silvet, M.D., who assisted me in my research and offered many useful suggestions for improving the manuscript. The reviewers also gave wonderful and detailed suggestions, for which I am very grateful. Special thanks to Robin Carter, Gina Wright, and Kerri Rabbitt, who were very patient in guiding me and were tolerant during delays, particularly after the death of my father.

Contents in Brief

Contents

1 | Triage: Critical Skills, Complexities, and Challenges

DEFINING TRIAGE: A DYNAMIC PROCESS

Triage involves the sorting of injured and ill persons into categories that prioritize them for medical care according to the nature and severity of their injury or illness. Determination of a patient's acuity is based on the patient's complaint and history, signs and symptoms, general appearance, vital signs, and the physical appraisal (Box 1–1).

The categories into which patients may be triaged for care include immediate (STAT), emergent, urgent, and nonurgent. "Levels" may be used in some systems for indicating the patient's acuity, typically level 1, 2, 3, or 4. Some facilities may use only three levels of acuity in triage: nonurgent, urgent, and emergent, and these are the descriptors that will be used in this book when discussing triage guidelines (Box 1–2).

Some facilities have developed guidelines, or algorithms, with specific factors that determine whether a patient's condition is "urgent" or "emergent." Intuition and judgment are critical factors in determining a patient's acuity level, and an algorithmic approach cannot account for these expert skills. Patients sometimes arrive at the emergency department (ED) with

---

BOX 1–1 | **Triage Acuity Determinants**

- Chief complaint
- Brief triage history
- Injury or illness (signs and symptoms)
- General appearance
- Vital signs
- Brief physical appraisal in triage

BOX 1–2	**Triage Acuity Levels**

- Nonurgent: Patient may safely wait for a long period to be seen or triaged for care to a clinic or primary health care provider.
- Urgent: Patient must be seen in the emergency department and should be reevaluated during the waiting period.
- Emergent: Patient should be triaged into the emergency department for care without delay because of the acuity of the injury or illness and the increased risk for loss of life or profound disability if waiting is required.

atypical symptoms or vague complaints that at first may not seem serious. However, the experienced triage nurse often discovers subtle signs of a serious health problem, even during the brief period when a patient is in the triage area. Triage cannot be operationalized in such a way that just anyone can safely perform this critical duty; it requires in-depth knowledge and experience.

An effective triage nurse relies on three fundamental skills when triaging patients: assessment, knowledge, and intuition. Although brief, triage assessments are systematic and consistent. Assessment always includes a brief patient history, clinical measurements, and a rapid, problem-oriented physical evaluation. Knowledge of mechanisms of injury, injury assessment, and a wide range of disease processes is essential to prioritize patients appropriately. Professionals who excel in triage use the skill of intuition. Intuition takes time to develop and requires a true interest in the process of triaging patients. Intuition is a "sixth sense" that helps determine the urgency of a patient's condition, as well as the frequency of reassessment and type of treatment. Intuition develops with experience, sensitivity, and the use of an observing eye that takes note of patients' presentation patterns. Intuition enables a triage nurse to put the picture together efficiently and quickly; it is a widely used and respected skill.

The role of the triage nurse is defined by the institution and

BOX 1–3	**Emergency Department Standards of Triage Care**

- Legal aspects of triage
- Critical skills for problem recognition and treatment
- Documentation
- Levels of triage
- Reassessment in the waiting area
- Dealing with behavioral and violent emergencies
- Resources for families needing consultation and assistance from other members of the health care team (e.g., social worker, police department, or other law enforcement or community agencies) should be reviewed with the triage nurse; clearly stated policies and resources must be readily available to the triage nurse.

department that regulate the position. Standards of care for triage in EDs are listed in Box 1–3.

Common responsibilities of the triage nurse in the ED are identified in Box 1–4.

TRIAGE SKILLS
Assessment

Assessment in triage is a two-tier process. In a setting where multiple patients require attention of the triage nurse, a rapid initial assessment takes place within 60 seconds of the patient's arrival at the triage area. This rapid assessment generally involves asking the patient (or the patient's designated historian, e.g., parent or friend) why medical care is being sought. Those who need immediate assessment include patients with airway compromise; cardiac complaints; injuries involving threat to life, limb, or neurologic integrity; traumatic and violent events such as child abuse or rape; or acutely dangerous psychoses (Box 1–5).

The art of triage in a busy situation requires tact, quickness, and an ability to communicate succinctly and with compassion. While patients' injuries and illnesses are often considered "minor" by professionals, it is important to keep in mind that to the patient, even a simple laceration can be traumatic. Fur-

BOX 1–4	**Responsibilities of the Triage Nurse**

- Initial inquiry to determine the patient's reason for seeking care
- Pretriage priority identification (In busy emergency departments the triage nurse decides the order in which arriving patients are officially triaged.)
- Triage history and assessment and documentation
- Triage designation
- Triage first aid, comfort measures, and fever care
- Orientation of the patient to the waiting room and expected time of wait until ED evaluation and care
- Communication with families and visitors regarding patient status in the ED when they are not allowed to visit
- Control and monitoring of the safety of the waiting area
- Reassessment and retriage of patients during the waiting period
- Telephone triage and phone communication with primary health care providers and insurance representatives if necessary
- Telephone communication as deemed appropriate with family members of patients requesting family notification
- Telephone communication with social services and law enforcement if required by institutional policy
- Referral of "nonurgent" patients meeting ED criteria to alternative facilities for care per agency policy
- Requests per ED protocols for initial laboratory and x-ray studies
- Writing of nursing orders for ED care per department protocols (e.g., reevaluation of blood pressure, patient education)
- Health education of patients and families as time permits
- Assistance of grieving family members and provision of private waiting area and help with basic needs if possible (e.g., tissues, water, and directions to restroom)

thermore, the triage nurse should never assume that a patient's injury or illness is minor based on the initial presentation. In a study of trauma patients done over a 3-year period at one level I trauma facility, researchers identified the following causes of provider-related complications, which triage nurses should consider: insensitivity of field triage protocols, inadequate recognition of injury patterns, and inadequate recognition of injury severity by providers (Hoyt et al., 1994). Triage nurses place

BOX 1–5	**Some Conditions Requiring Immediate Triage**

- Airway compromise
- Cardiac complaints
- Injuries involving threat to life or limb
- Critical neurologic problems (e.g., altered level of consciousness)
- Violent traumas (e.g., child abuse, domestic violence, and rape)
- Dangerous psychoses or patients with a potential for harming themselves or others
- Poisoning
- Anaphylaxis
- Hypoglycemia or hyperglycemia
- Critical burns

potential trauma patients at risk for complications if the nurses do not thoroughly but quickly assess individuals who meet criteria that identify them as qualifying for entry into the trauma system.

Many of the patients visiting the ED for primary health care and emergencies are adolescents. One study of 11 counties in California demonstrated that of 10,493 prehospital care report forms, adolescents (ages 12 to 18 years) required prehospital care and ED care more frequently than any other pediatric age-group (Seidel, 1991). Parental consent is not required for treatment of any medical emergency, sexually transmissible diseases, or pregnancy or for drug or alcohol abuse services (Selbst, 1985). Parents and legal guardians should also be contacted whenever possible unless it is unsafe for the child, but the triage nurse should not hesitate to begin the triage process in the absence of a parent or guardian if the child meets the aforementioned criteria. Furthermore, in many states minors may seek care independently, without permission of their legal guardian, if they are "emancipated." Examples of qualifying conditions for emancipation may include being married (previously or at present); being a high school graduate, pregnant (previously or at present), or self-supporting; serving in the armed forces; living independently; being a runaway; or having been abandoned (Selbst, 1985). The triage nurse must be familiar with state laws, and triage policies must reflect state and federal laws that pertain to pediatric patients.

Patient History

Once a patient has the full attention of a triage professional, a minimal assessment is performed to determine which triage cat-

---

| BOX 1–6 | **Triage History** |

IDENTIFYING DATA

Name, age, sex, primary language, mode of transportation, accompanying persons

CHIEF COMPLAINT

Reason for seeking care (stated in the patient's own words if possible)

PRESENT ILLNESS

When chief complaint began or when it occurred, nature of problem at present, efforts to control problem, and results

ALLERGIES TO MEDICATIONS

Including symptoms of allergic response

MEDICATIONS

Including type, dosage, frequency, last dose, and compliance

PRIMARY HEALTH CARE PROVIDER

Name and last visit

LAST MENSTRUAL PERIOD

Record first day of LMP
Gravidity, parity, abortions (spontaneous or induced). If vaginal bleeding: number of pads or tampons per hour or day, number of days or hours since bleeding started

TETANUS HISTORY

All-vaccine status for pediatric patients

HOME REMEDIES AND ALTERNATIVE HEALTH MEASURES USED AND RESPONSE

---

egory is most appropriate for the patient (Box 1–6). History information obtained from the patient should include chief complaint, the time the problem began (illness) or occurred (injury), and the nature of the problem at present. Associated symptoms and attempts to control the problem before arriving at the triage area are recorded, and information regarding allergies, medications (including time, type, dosage, and last dose—both prescription and nonprescription), primary health care provider, last tetanus booster, last menstrual period, and number of pregnancies, deliveries, and abortions (spontaneous and induced).

If a patient is accompanied by another person, that person's relationship to the patient is recorded. It is also helpful to know whether the friend or family member has provided transportation for the patient. The triage professional should make a note regarding the patient's state of orientation.

Triage Examination

The triage assessment continues as the patient's vital signs are obtained and a cursory problem-specific or system-specific examination is performed (Box 1–7). Because of the time lag between triage and treatment, first aid may be performed concurrently with triage. Laceration characteristics are evaluated (location and extent) and recorded, and interventions to control bleeding and minimize the potential for infection are instituted. Fever-control measures such as oral or rectal administration of acetaminophen may be instituted in triage depending on the patient's history of allergies and what medications have already been used to control fever or discomfort at home (Fig. 1–1).

BOX 1–7 | **Triage Physical Assessment Data**

- Clinical measurements: vital signs and weight
- Limited orthostatics: Pulse and blood pressure, both sitting and standing (indicate arm used)
- Evaluation for peripheral vascular integrity
- Injury examination
- Measurement of pupils

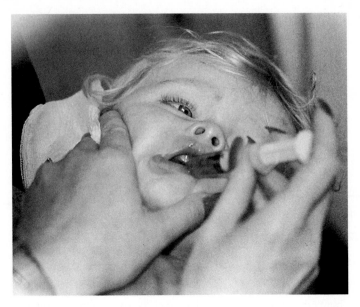

Fig. 1–1 Acetaminophen administration during triage is an appropriate intervention for febrile patients.

Objective Assessment Data

In addition to obtaining history information and performing an initial physical examination on patients, triage nurses in some hospitals are assigned minimal laboratory duties to more accurately determine the patient's acuity and to decide what area of the ED is most appropriate for the patient's needs. These duties may include obtaining a urine sample and evaluating it for blood and/or white blood cell (WBC) count with dipstick, performing rapid urine pregnancy tests, and obtaining blood for a spun hematocrit or a rapid blood sugar analysis (Fig. 1–2). A patient's oxygen saturation as determined by pulse oximetry is another example of objective data that may be obtained by the triage nurse. Obtaining laboratory data is optional in that it requires that sufficient support personnel be available. Box 1–8 summarizes objective data that may be obtained in triage.

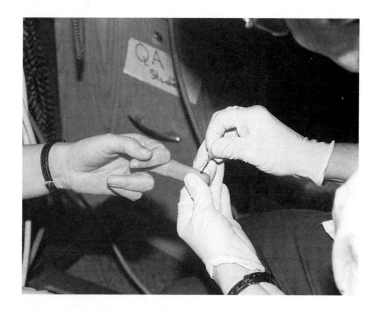

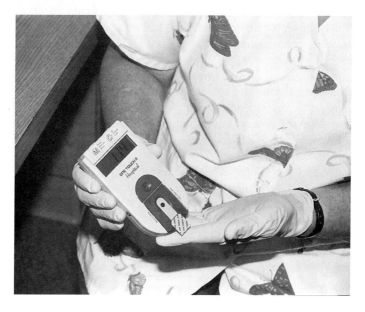

Fig. 1–2 Rapid blood sugar assessment can assist in triage.

BOX 1–8	Objective Triage Data

- Urine analysis by dipstick (e.g., for white or red blood cells or bacteria)
- Vision (Snellen or Rosenbaum chart)
- Pulse oximetry before oxygen therapy unless the patient regularly uses oxygen (record which)
- Glucometer blood sugar analysis
- Rapid urine pregnancy testing
- Spun hematocrit
- Peak flow (forced expiratory volume)

Knowledge

Effective triage depends on the nurse's ability to make a rapid yet thorough assessment. The initial history and physical assessment in triage, however brief, vary according to the nurse's suspicion about what the problem may be. In all situations the ABCs (airway, breathing, and circulation) must be assessed. Airway patency is determined by establishing that the patient exhibits no signs or symptoms of respiratory compromise related to airway integrity (e.g., stridor or cyanosis). Breathing should be eupneic, as determined by normal respiratory rate, rhythm, and depth; evidence of equal chest expansion; and the absence of respiratory distress signs and symptoms (e.g., use of accessory muscles or nasal flaring). Circulation integrity is assessed in triage by obtaining the patient's pulse and blood pressure. Obtaining an apical pulse may be necessary if the patient's peripheral radial pulse is weak, irregular, bradycardic, or tachycardic. Blood pressure must be measured using a blood pressure cuff appropriate for the age and size of the patient (Fig. 1–3). Manual (rather than electronic) assessment tools are consistently accurate and should be available. If electronic tools are used, they should initially be calibrated with manual tools. Knowledge of the basic elements of injury and illness assessment is necessary. These elements are best categorized according to chief complaints for medical-surgical problems and for injuries by mechanism of injury.

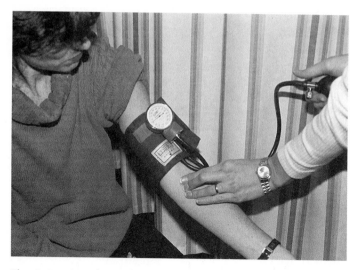

Fig. 1–3 A pediatric blood pressure cuff may be necessary for adult patients with small arms.

BOX 1–9	**Triage Questions Related to Mechanisms of Injury**

- What happened?
- Where exactly were you when the accident occurred?
- What did you see, hear, smell, feel?
- What was the first thing you did after the accident?
- What have you done to treat your injuries since the accident occurred?

Patients must be questioned about when an injury occurred or when an illness began. Further details are needed depending on the chief complaint. Patients who have had an injury need to be asked about the mechanism of the injury; their answer may cue the examine to consider internal trauma (Box 1–9).

Questions to ask patients who have suffered a motor vehicle accident (MVA) are listed in Box 1–10. Specific examples

BOX 1–10	**Triage Questions Related to Motor Vehicle Accidents**

- When did the accident happen? (day and time)
- Where did it occur? (freeway, street) This information enables health care providers to estimate probable speed of the vehicle during the accident and to understand which law enforcement agency should be contacted about the accident.
- What was your position in the vehicle? (driver or passenger, and if passenger, exactly where in the vehicle) This information enables the health care provider to understand possible forces that may have impacted the patient during the accident.
- Did you lose consciousness? If so, for how long, and what are the first and last things you remember?
- Were you wearing a seatbelt? If so, what type? (lap belt or shoulder harness or both) Was it effective during the accident?
- Does your car have an airbag? If so, where? Did the airbag inflate on impact?
- How were you injured in the accident? Did a flying object, such as another person, hit you? Did you slam up against the door?
- Did you hear anything in association with your injuries? (e.g., a pop or crack)
- How fast were you going? If another car was involved, do you know how fast the other car was going?
- What happened to the vehicle? What kind of vehicle was it? (type, especially, is helpful, e.g., small car, truck, or motorcycle)
- Were you ejected from the vehicle? Were you extricated or assisted out?
- Were there others in the accident who were severely injured or killed?

of what to ask when individuals have suffered near-drowning, falls, or sharp trauma such as stab wounds are given in Chapter 3, under events, and in Chapters 6 through 12, which deal with system-specific patient complaints.

Triage criteria related to presentations of accidents, injuries, or symptoms that require that a case be designated as a ''trauma'' are included in Box 1–11. A patient designated as a

BOX 1–11	**Mechanisms of Injury and Trauma Designation**

TRAUMA DESIGNATION

Major codes

Full arrest after traumatic event (triage nurse responds to parking lot/drive-up trauma)

Proximal amputations

Penetrating wounds to the head or torso-to-knee level (elbows in and knees up)

Death of an occupant in the same vehicle

CRAMS scale score ≤8 and Glasgow Coma Scale ≤12

Motorcycle accident with injury

Auto versus pedestrian accident

Ejection from vehicle

Death of occupant in the other vehicle

CONSIDERATION FOR TRAUMA DESIGNATION

Minor codes

CRAMS scale score of 9 or 10

Patients older than 65 years with major injuries (excluding falls and fractured hips)

Falls of more than 12 feet

Near-drowning with cervical spine involvement, such as diving injuries (otherwise a medical code)

Burns (based on CRAMS scale score) and potential for other injuries (e.g., in the event of an explosion)

Hangings (cervical spine involvement)

---

trauma patient is automatically classified as requiring ''emergent'' care and is triaged into the trauma room or trauma system without delay. Further assessment that would normally be done in the triage area, such as obtaining vital signs, is done in the trauma area or resuscitation area in facilities that are not trauma centers. The criteria for trauma are being continually reevaluated. Because of the high cost of delivering trauma care and maintaining trauma facilities, reevaluation is appropriately ongoing in an effort to specifically determine which patients need to receive immediate care from an ED and which patients will be likely to survive and do well only with the full range of services provided by a trauma center.

DeKeyser et al. (1994) reported a two-tier system for trauma whereby two distinct teams are initiated, depending on the trauma patient's acuity. This system has saved their institution $629,404 per year from reduced use of personnel, protective clothing, and services.

Patients who are injured are scored on the CRAMS scale (Box 1–12), a universally accepted assessment tool that is useful

---

BOX 1–12   CRAMS Scale

CIRCULATION

Normal capillary refill and BP > 100	2
Delayed capillary refill or BP 85–100	1
No capillary refill or BP < 85	0

RESPIRATION

Normal	2
Abnormal (labored or shallow)	1
Absent	0

ABDOMEN

Abdomen and thorax nontender	2
Abdomen or thorax tender	1
Abdomen rigid, flail chest, or penetrating wounds to abdomen or thorax	0

MOTOR

Normal	2
Responds only to pain (other than decerebrate)	1
No response (or decerebrate)	0

SPEECH

Normal	2
Confused	1
No intelligible words	0
TOTAL SCORE =	10

---

in determining the severity of the patient's condition and the prognosis. The patient should be assessed for a CRAMS score initially by either the triage nurse or the ED nurse if the patient has been brought immediately into the department and then on a periodic basis. The acuity level of a patient should not be based on the CRAMS score because the triage nurse must judge the patient's acuity on the basis of the chief complaint, physical assessment, general appearance, and objective data. The CRAMS score is an objective tool that provides a measurable baseline, which can be useful, in part, for determining the degree of progress or deterioration a patient exhibits once treatment has ensued or during evaluations subsequent to the initial triage assessment.

The Champion is a trauma scoring scale used to determine the patient's level of acuity and prognosis. Because it is more extensive in categories and is deemed by many to not be ''user friendly,'' it is not as universally implemented as a scoring tool as the CRAMS scale is. In relation to trauma, a pediatric trauma score (PTS) was studied by Kaufmann et al. (1990) to determine whether it was more helpful than traditional scoring methods for trauma, such as the CRAMS scale. Use of the PTS was not recommended, since it was found to be less accurate and required field and hospital personnel to learn a separate scoring system for triaging patients (Kaufmann et al., 1990). An abdominal injury trauma score being evaluated for use in pediatric patients is showing promise in predicting the risk of abdominal injury in children after blunt trauma (Box 1–13). Based on the child's score, a risk category of low, intermediate, or high is assigned, and the score is used in conjunction with clinical judgment to determine the need for radiographic studies of the abdomen, such as computerized laparotomy (Taylor et al., 1994). This score may be useful in pediatric EDs where a high concentration of children is served.

A commonly used scale in triage and ED care is the Glasgow Coma Scale (Box 1–14). This scale is used to determine neurologic integrity. The Glasgow Coma Scale should be used on patients with head trauma or neurologic complaints (e.g., severe sudden-onset headache or syncope). As with the CRAMS scale, the Glasgow Coma Scale provides an objective tool that is a useful part of the patient's baseline assessment

BOX 1–13	**Abdominal Injury Score**

VARIABLE	PARTIAL SCORE
Mechanism of injury	
Motor vehicle accident (MVA) passenger	4
MVA, pedestrian	8
Fall	15
Bicycle accident	15
Abuse or assault	12
Lap belt	24
Other	0
Trauma score <12	10
Abdominal tenderness	12
Absent bowel sounds	5
Fractured pelvis	10
Gross hematuria	14
Chest trauma	7
Hematocrit value <30%	9
TOTAL SCORE*	
Low risk, >14	
Intermediate risk, 15–26	
High risk, >26	

Modified from Taylor G et al: *Radiology* 190(3):689, 1994.
*Total score is the summation of the partial scores for whichever variables are present.

against which the patient is reevaluated by other health care providers.

The accuracy of the Glasgow Coma Scale may be affected if the patient is hypoxic or hypotensive; thus it is important to highlight the presence of these symptoms so that other health care personnel will consider the patient's Glasgow Coma Scale score in light of the overall presentation. A reevaluation of the accuracy of the Glasgow Coma Scale in critically ill or injured patients has been recommended, and the use of alternative scoring systems for neurologic assessment has been considered (Marion and Carlier, 1994).

BOX 1–14	Glasgow Coma Scale

EYE OPENING

Spontaneous	4
To voice	3
To pain	2
None	1

VERBAL RESPONSE

Oriented	5
Confused	4
Inappropriate words	3
Incomprehensible words	2
None	1

MOTOR RESPONSE

Obeys command	6
Localizes pain	5
Withdraws (pain)	4
Flexion (pain)	3
Extension (pain)	2
None	1
TOTAL SCORE (MAXIMUM)	15

Intuition

Intuition is a little-studied yet widely used skill of the triage nurse. Intuition is a ''sixth sense'' that a patient is having a particular problem, is at risk for certain problems or complications, or needs particular attention to a symptom or set of symptoms. At times an experienced triage nurse who evaluates a patient finds that, although the history may be vague and the vital signs and presentation relatively unremarkable, the nurse has a ''feeling'' that something critical is about to go wrong. Often the patient's condition is then designated as emergent rather than nonurgent or urgent, and several minutes later that patient ''codes'' or has a seizure, or in some way exhibits problems that require immediate therapy. The unexplained sense that allowed the triage nurse to enter the patient into the ED as an "emergent" patient is based not in the "cosmos" but rather on experience, observation of multiple patients with varying problems and presentations over a period of years, knowledge of diseases and injuries, and conversations held with other health care providers from the ED and other specialty areas regarding patterns of presentations noticed during triage and evaluation of patients. There is a need for ongoing research in this area to validate the value of intuition and to study factors that promote its development.

Facilitating the Appropriate Use of Emergency Services

Visits to EDs in 1990 increased nationwide 19% from 85 million to 99 million, during which time inpatient admissions decreased by 7%. The greatest increase in ED usage was seen in patients with Medicaid and Medicare coverage. It is estimated that in 1990, 43% of patients had injuries or illnesses that could have been treated in less expensive settings if they had been accessible (Policy: use of emergency departments, 1993). The increase in ED usage is probably a result of many factors, including lack of available nonemergency services and lack of information on how to access primary or urgent care providers.

A shortage of community resources and lack of awareness of how to access available services are often the root causes for indigent patients' seeking primary care services from the ED. Pane et al. (1991) found that at the University of California–Irvine Medical Center ED, which treats an average of 38,000 patients per year, "low-income individuals and those with public aid or self-pay insurance status were significantly more likely to use the ED as a routine source of health care, and more likely to delay in seeking needed health care, than higher income and fully insured individuals." Use of the ED to receive primary health care is inappropriate but often unavoidable. This issue should be addressed by EDs, community agencies, and representatives in the community. If cooperation exists between community clinics and EDs, triaging patients to area clinics may be an option. Derlet et al. (1992) reported that in their 3-year study, 21,069 (15%) of 136,794 patients were triaged away from the ED to receive services elsewhere without any major adverse effects as determined by follow-up calls to the area clinics, EDs, and coroners' offices. In an earlier study by Derlet and Nishio (1991), 4186 patients were triaged out in the first 6 months of the new policy to triage out patients with nonurgent problems; not only was this found to be safe (there were no major adverse outcomes), but only 54 (1.3%) of the patients complained about their referral to alternative services.

Triaging to area clinics and health care facilities is ideal for the ''nonurgent'' patient because primary care can be delivered in a setting where follow-up and continuity of care are possible (i.e., the same provider who gives initial care also evaluates the effectiveness of the treatment over time). This practice also reduces the waiting time for patients who truly require emergency services. It is cost-effective for all concerned and should be used not only for indigent patients but also for those with primary health care providers who have the ability to see the patient in a timely manner.

Guidelines for nonemergency complaints that may be triaged for care outside the ED must be clearly defined and not too broad in scope. Lowe et al. (1994) report that 51 nonemergency complaints that were identified for ''triage out'' would have resulted in a 33% margin of error. Of the 106 patients who would have met nonemergency criteria for being triaged out, 4 were hospitalized. The authors rightly concluded that *broad application* of the guidelines would jeopardize the health of some patients.

STRATEGIES TO MAXIMIZE RESOURCES

Excessive waiting periods for patients are often caused by an imbalance between supply of and demand for beds. Long waiting periods for patients with complaints that need professional evaluation and treatment can lead to patients' leaving without being seen by a health care professional. This may result in serious consequences. Baker et al. (1991) studied 186 patients in a public hospital ED who, during a 2-week period, left the ED without receiving attention. Of these patients, 46% were judged to need immediate medical attention, 29% needed care within 24 to 48 hours, 11% were hospitalized within the next week, and 3 patients required emergency surgery. The researchers concluded that excessive waiting times (6.4 hours on average in this report) restrict access to care for the poor and uninsured. This finding is particularly significant when the reasons that patients left—problems with transportation, baby-sitting, or work schedules—are considered. In another study, 15% of patients waited a median of 3 hours but up to 17 hours to be seen and left without being seen by a physician, and 4% of the patients required subsequent hospitalization, with 27% returning to an ED (Bindman et al., 1991). The solution to over-crowding of EDs begins by studying the use of EDs. Rask et al. (1994), in a study of 3897 patients seeking ED care, found that 48.4% of the 2341 patients with a new medical problem delayed seeking health care for more than 2 days because of having no health insurance or no transportation, fearing exposure to vio-lence, or living in a supervised setting.

Education below high-school level is also positively cor-related with delay in seeking health care. While some patients use EDs for primary health care, those with serious or new med-ical problems sometimes have increased morbidity and mor-tality as a result of waiting too long to have their problems evaluated; this increases cost and reduces success in treatment. Recommendations that patients use urgent-care community cen-ters or ambulatory care sites may be of limited help if the sites do not provide access to care for Medicaid or self-pay patients. In a study of 953 ambulatory care sites, researchers found that access to care is severely limited because of inconvenient or short hours of operation and unwillingness to treat patients with Medicaid. The researchers conclude, "Medicaid recipients in urban areas have limited access to outpatient care apart from that offered by hospital emergency departments" (Access of Medicaid recipients to outpatient care, 1994).

Alleviating overcrowding in the ED can be accomplished through triaging "nonurgent" patients to area clinics and health care providers, by developing a "fast track" within the ED to handle simple cases such as simple lacerations or earaches, and by developing an observation unit to monitor patients who need continued nursing and medical care but who may not need to be admitted to the hospital (e.g., patients with uncomplicated chest pain or asthmatics requiring inhalation therapies). Work to prevent patient problems within the community (e.g., poison control and pollution alerts) is also helpful in alleviating over-crowding by addressing the problems that affect many patients.

Evaluation of Patterns of Emergency Department Use

Strategies for preventive and primary care outside the ED must be developed to make health care more accessible for all in a cost-effective manner. Investing in preventing ED misuse by patients of low socioeconomic status can be particularly cost-effective for hospitals that serve the underprivileged. These patients frequently require more resources and hospitalization than patients of higher socioeconomic status (Stern et al., 1991). Partnerships between ED personnel and public health departments, school health personnel, and other community agencies should be developed to educate the community on the signs, symptoms, and treatment of common illnesses. Regardless of race and socioeconomic status, many patients with minor illnesses believe that medical problems should be evaluated by a health care provider within 24 hours and use the ED for health care because of its easy access and the wide range of services offered (Shesser et al., 1991). Educating the community about the purpose of the ED and alternatives for health care—as well as developing careful, safe policies for "triaging out" patients with minor health problems, particularly adults—may reduce the cost of ED use for minor health problems. Emergency departments should also study and address the special needs of the elderly, since this population is increasing in the United States and its use of EDs for emergent health care is also increasing (Singal et al., 1992).

Urgent Care Areas or "Fast Tracks"

Federal estimates of ED use by patients with nonurgent problems indicate that between 40% and 55% of all ED visits involve nonurgent problems (Kellermann, 1994). "Fast track" or urgent care units within EDs have been developed in many facilities to handle patients with nonurgent complaints. Wright et al. (1992) reported that 28% of 4468 patients who sought medical attention at the authors' ED were triaged to a nurse practitioner–staffed fast track in the first year of its operation, that fewer than 1% of patients required admission to the hospital, and that, on average, the total ED time was 94.4 minutes. General Hospital Medical Center in Everett, Washington, found a reduction in waiting time for 30% of their patients—from a waiting time of 90 to 150 minutes to a consistent 90-minute waiting time—from triage to discharge when a fast track unit was opened for defined noncritical problems (Romanelli, 1992). Protocols and standing orders were developed, which enhanced the rapid evaluation and treatment of specified problems. Problems that may be considered appropriate for fast track treatment are listed in Box 1–15.

Nursing managers must avoid using an urgent care or fast track area for acute care overflow. Urgent care areas are not typically equipped with everything necessary for safe nursing care of patients with acute problems. These areas are also staffed with a lower nurse-to-patient ratio, and there may be insufficient staff to care for acutely ill patients. For a disaster or an unusual situation when urgent care beds must be used for overflow, the area must be staffed sufficiently with nurses to provide safe care for ill and injured patients who require close attention and definitive care.

Fast tracks in some EDs may have a specific definition and function whereby patients with classified and acute problems such as myocardial infarction are handled in a rapid, definitive manner. This is a form of secondary triage. In one unit 359 myocardial infarction (MI) patients (who met clinical and electrocardiographic criteria) were given rapid access to a cardiac care team, bypassing usual emergency medical evaluation. This secondary rapid triage of MI patients for care resulted in a dramatic reduction in delay of thrombolytic therapy for those re-

---

BOX 1–15	**Fast Track Candidates**

- Corneal abrasions
- Conjunctivitis
- Earache
- Toothache
- Puncture wound
- Minor laceration
- Minor head trauma (without loss of consciousness)

quiring it and more rapid and efficient admission to the cardiac care unit (Pell et al., 1992). Recognition that the fast track concept is useful in secondary triage demonstrates that this concept is a timesaving, sensible approach to treating emergency patients.

Observation Units

Observation units are in use in large hospitals to provide nursing care for ED patients who require observation and medical treatment but who probably will not require admission within a 24-hour period. Eagle (1991) reported on a protocol for determining which patients with cardiac-related complaints can be monitored for a 12-hour period in an observation unit versus a prolonged evaluation period in an intensive care unit (ICU). Patients in this study who were selected for an observation approach rather than ICU observation had a low rate of complications.

Both observation and fast track units are helpful in freeing ED beds for patients needing emergency services.

ECONOMIC FACTORS AFFECTING TRIAGE

Triage nurses who are instructed to request information about insurance or financial matters are operating outside the realm of triage nursing. Eliciting financial information should be the function of a clerk after the patient has been evaluated by the nurse. In this age of managed care and health maintenance organizations (HMOs) the agreement of an insurance company to pay for a visit to the ED is of great concern to the patient; however, the physical health and safety of the individual are paramount and are the legal responsibility of the health care providers in the ED. It is dangerous for patients to be refused services based on their inability to pay or based on the lack of agreement by the insurance company to pay. When a patient has had the advantage of an initial evaluation by a professional nurse and has been assigned a triage category, determination of where the patient can best be cared for can be made in a safe, helpful manner.

Triage nurses may choose to act as advocates for patients in the event that an insurance company refuses to authorize payment for a patient to be seen in the ED; if this occurs, documentation of this action should be charted, including the outcome and the insurance representative's name. The assumption should not be made that HMO insurance will not approve ED evaluation or hospital admission. In a study of 3006 patients entering an ED with chest pain who were considered a medium to low risk for acute MI, investigators found that HMO membership was associated with higher rates of hospital admission (Pearson et al., 1994). The triage nurse must always keep an open mind when she/he deals with insurance companies.

Department Policies and Triage

Triage nurses should be well informed regarding the principles of the American College of Emergency Physicians for emergency care of patients. These principles should be consistent with triage policies and guidelines. The principles relevant to triage are summarized in Box 1–16.

Policies that apply to triage should be periodically reviewed, with input welcomed from medicine, nursing, volunteer services, and a representative from the general public who can

---

BOX 1–16	**Principles of Emergency Care Endorsed by the American College of Emergency Physicians**

- All patients presenting to an ED with an emergency medical condition should receive an appropriate medical evaluation and stabilization by emergency physicians and/or consultant physicians in a timely manner and without consideration of ability to pay for these services.
- Patients who come to the ED to be evaluated by their private physician should be offered an appropriate evaluation if their private physician is not available in the ED in a timely manner.
- The hospital and its medical staff are responsible for providing or ensuring access to appropriate consulting, admitting, and follow-up physicians for all ED patients. Such physicians must be available in a timely manner, without regard to the ability of the patient to pay for these services.

Modified from American College of Emergency Physicians: *Ann Emerg Med* 22(11):1787, 1993.

speak from the patient's perspective. Policies that are not helpful in triage include policies indicating that patients are triaged on a "first-come, first-served" basis and policies that routinely bar families from access to their loved ones who are being treated in the ED.

The Evolving Nature of Triage

It often seems that when one begins discussing an intimate problem with a patient, another patient rushes in with acute chest pain and the first patient must be cleared out of the triage area so that the patient with the more acute condition can be evaluated. To reduce the embarrassment and discomfort patients may face, it is importance to orient each patient to the purpose and process of triage. This orientation clarifies the brevity of the interview, introduces the possibility that the process may be interrupted, and facilitates cooperation.

Interruptions in triage can significantly reduce the efficiency of the triage nurse and greatly increase the pretriage waiting time for patients who require medical attention. Interruptions may include handling telephone triage duties and tending to non-triage-related requests. The number of interruptions and length of time patients wait in the pretriage period have been significantly correlated in one study of triage implementation (Geraci and Geraci, 1994). Use of ancillary personnel such as volunteers to assist in non-triage-related functions may increase the efficiency of triage nurses and decrease the pretriage waiting period for patients.

The effectiveness of triage is evaluated by means of the ED's quality assurance program with attention to the following: sufficient documentation in determination of acuity level, adequate charting of patient complaints and symptoms, identity of the historian during charting (such as the patient, parent, or significant other), and duration or onset of illness or accident charted (*California Emergency Nurse Newsletter,* 1992).

REFERENCES

Access of Medicaid recipients to outpatient care, *N Engl J Med* 330(20):1426, 1994.
American College of Emergency Physicians: Medical staff responsi-

bility for emergency department patients, *Ann Emerg Med* 22(11):1787, 1993.

Baker D, Stevens C, Brook R: Patients who leave a public hospital emergency department without being seen by a physician: causes and consequences, *JAMA* 266(8):1085, 1991.

Bindman AB et al: Consequences of cueing for care at a public hospital emergency department, *JAMA* 266(8):1091, 1991.

California Emergency Nurse Newsletter, vol 9, summer 1992.

DeKeyser F et al: Decreasing the cost of trauma care: a system of secondary in hospital triage, *Ann Emerg Med* 23(4):841, 1994.

Derlet R, Nishio D: Refusing care to patients who present to an emergency department, *Ann Emerg Med* 19(3):262, 1990.

Derlet R et al: Triage of patients out of the emergency department: three-year experience, *Am J Emerg Med* 10(3):195, 1992.

Eagle K: Medical decision making in patients with chest pain, *N Engl J Med* 324(18): 1282, 1991.

Geraci E, Geraci T: An observational study of the emergency triage nursing role in a managed care facility, *J Emerg Nurs* 20(3):189, 1994.

Hoyt D et al: Analysis of recurrent process errors leading to provider-related complications on an organized trauma service: directions for care improvement, *J Trauma* 36(3):377, 1994.

Kaufmann CR et al: Evaluation of the Pediatric Trauma Score, *JAMA* 263(1):69, 1990.

Kellermann A: Nonurgent emergency department visits: meeting an unmet need, *JAMA* 271(24):1953, 1994 (editorial comment).

Lowe R et al: Refusing care to emergency department patients: evaluation of published triage guidelines, *Ann Emerg Med* 23(2):286, 1994.

Marion D, Carlier P: Problems with initial Glasgow Coma Scale assessment caused by prehospital treatment of patients with head injuries: results of a national survey, *J Trauma* 36(1):89, 1994.

Pane G, Farner M, Salness K: Health care access problems of medically indigent emergency department walk-in patients, *Ann Emerg Med* 20(7):730, 1991.

Pearson S et al: The impact of membership in a health maintenance organization on hospital admission rates for acute chest pain, *Health Serv Res* 29(1):59, 1994.

Pell A et al: Effect of "fast track" admission for acute myocardial infarction on delay to thrombolysis, *Br Med J* 304(6819):83, 1992.

Policy: use of emergency departments, *Hospitals* 67(4):14, 1993 (news).

Rask K et al: Obstacles predicting lack of a regular provider and delays in seeking care for patients at an urban public hospital, *JAMA* 271(24):1931, 1994.

Romanelli N: We put ED patients on the fast track, *RN* 55(7):17, 20, 1992.

Seidel J: Emergency medical services and the adolescent patient, *J Adolesc Health* 12(2):95, 1991.

Selbst S: Treating minors without their parents, *Pediatr Emerg Care* 1:168, 1985.

Shesser R et al: An analysis of emergency department use by patients with minor illness, *Ann Emerg Med* 20(7):743, 1991.

Singal B et al: Geriatric patient emergency visits. Part I. Comparison of visits by geriatric and younger patients, *Ann Emerg Med* 21(7):802, 1992.

Stern R, Weissman J, Epstein A: The emergency department as a pathway to admission for poor and high-cost patients, *JAMA* 266(16):2238, 1991.

Taylor G et al: Abdominal injury score: a clinical score for the assignment of risk in children after blunt trauma, *Radiology* 190(3):689, 1994.

Wright S et al: Fast track in the emergency department: a one-year experience with nurse practitioners, *J Emerg Med* 10(3): 367, 1992.

RECOMMENDED READING

American College of Emergency Physicians: Emergency care guidelines, *Ann Emerg Med* 20(12):646, 1993.

American College of Emergency Physicians: Medical staff responsibility for emergency department patients, *Ann Emerg Med* 22(11): 1787, 1993.

Baker D, Stevens C, Brook R: Regular source of ambulatory care and medical utilization by patients presenting to a public hospital emergency department, *JAMA* 271(24):1909, 1994.

Brown E, Sindelar J: The emergent problem of ambulance misuse, *Ann Emerg Med* 22(4):646, 1993.

Hoyt D et al: Analysis of recurrent process errors leading to provider-related complications on an organized trauma service: directions for care improvement, *J Trauma* 36(3):377, 1994.

Pearson S et al: The impact of membership in a health maintenance organization on hospital admission rates for acute chest pain, *Health Serv Res* 29(1):59, 1994.

Purnell L: A survey of the qualifications, special training, and level of personnel working emergency department triage, *J Staff Develop* 9(5):223, 1900.

Wrenn K et al: The use of structured, complaint-specific patient encounter forms in the emergency department, *Ann Emerg Med* 22(5):805, 1993.

2 | Triage Settings

Recommendations for triaging patients appropriately into the categories defined in Chapter 1, emergent, urgent, and nonurgent, are universal to all triage situations. Individuals who have an immediate threat to life or limb always have the highest priority for care except in a disaster situation, when resources and personnel are directed to care for those with the highest likelihood of survival.

While the implementation of triage policies should reflect an understanding of basic triage principles, variations in environments, personnel, and patient populations affect how well triaging works. Recognition of the unchanging features in the triage process is a necessary precedent to discussing the elements of triage that vary and require creative skills in order to be efficient and effective. Sorting ill and injured patients into priority categories through triaging is usually discussed in relation to emergency medicine, but it is relevant to office practice, school health, and any situation where health care is provided to individuals who need to be evaluated on a walk-in basis or who seek care without an appointment. It is imperative that standards be set for what aspects of assessment and care must always be incorporated or considered for every triage setting. In addition, unique environments that necessitate flexibility and creativity in decision making as it applies to triage must be discussed.

THE HUMAN RESPONSE TO TRAGEDY

One fundamental element in the triage process that rarely varies is the human response of the patient and bystanders to an accident or illness that causes the patient to require emergency services. The response of each individual to tragedy (whether minor or major in perception or reality) is dynamic and is controlled by several factors. The first factor is the individual's physiologic response to stress. This response is determined by the individual's perception of the level of threat the problem is causing, by the coping skills available to the individual, by past experiences with similar situations, and by the person's current state of general health and basic needs. Although it is not realistic for the triage nurse to assess the patient's and each family member's response to the tragedy, the triage nurse is responsible for the initial comfort of and communication with individuals affected by a crisis. Gentle touch, a concerned manner, and attention to basic comfort measures, such as offering a chair and a glass of water if appropriate, are often remembered with gratitude by patients and family members when they recall the initial response of the emergency department (ED) team to their situation. It has been said well by Lynne Gagnon (1991) that "those of us who work there every day may not realize how intimidating an ED environment can be for those who do not." Consideration for a patient's basic needs is a tangible way for triage nurses to always demonstrate concern.

Pediatric patients must be treated with consideration for the effects of psychologic stress on their physiologic health. It is important for the child to feel as relaxed and trusting as possible so that the overall consequences of stress resulting from the illness and the experience in the ED can be minimized (Thomas, 1991). Suggestions for providing a positive experience in triage are provided in Box 2–1.

When family members of injured patients approach the triage nurse, it is important to assess their physical stability and respond quickly if assistance, such as a wheelchair for an elderly spouse, is necessary.

When family members of a deceased patient arrive at the triage area, the triage nurse should be efficient in activating the bereavement team if one is available at the facility. If at all possible, bereaved relatives of a deceased patient should be taken to a private waiting area (Cooke et al., 1992) and provided with necessities for their comfort (such as tissues, water, and a telephone). The ED staff should be notified of the family's arrival so that the physician and nurse involved with the deceased patient's care can communicate directly with the family. A structured, multidisciplinary approach to bereavement is helpful in caring for the family of a deceased patient and significant

BOX 2–1	**Suggestions for Triage Success With Pediatric Patients**

- Treat the child with patience
- Talk directly to the child and be honest
- Be firm but kind, using gentle touch with warm hands
- Do not convey panic: Move swiftly if necessary but in a calm manner
- Allow the parents or those accompanying the child who are a comfort to stay with the child as much as possible (Fig. 2–1)
- Allow the child to make simple choices
- Be readily forthcoming with rewards such as stickers (Fig. 2–2)
- Do not embarrass the child by performing procedures that cause the body to be exposed in triage unless absolutely imperative

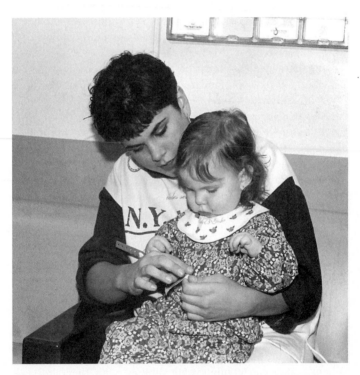

Fig. 2–1   Pediatric patients should be held by a parent for success in triage and comfort.

others and providing timely care and information (Adamowski et al, 1993). The triage nurse should be sensitive to the grief many patients of spontaneous abortion feel at the actual, impending, or threatened loss of the pregnancy, and comfort measures should be taken to alleviate such a patient's anguish whenever possible (Walters and Tupin, 1991).

The second factor influencing response to crisis is the individual's psychologic response to stress as determined by the perceived need to "be strong" and by how much permission the person feels to express or experience emotions. Many medics have witnessed the superhuman ability of mothers to respond to and care for their children's needs in accidents when they themselves have been critically injured. One cannot assume a patient's level of injury based on initial presentation alone. This is true not only in the field but in the triage area as well.

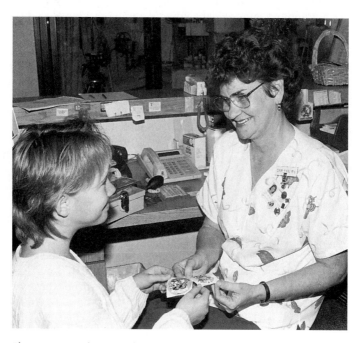

Fig. 2-2   Stickers can be effective rewards.

Triage nurses must be astutely aware that an individual's appearance of "coping well" with an injury or illness may be just that—a function of coping—and not an indication of the severity of his or her condition. An objective eye must be maintained throughout the brief history taking and assessment done in the triage area to accurately determine any patient's actual acuity level based on the history and a brief physical evaluation.

The third factor influencing response to crisis is the individual's sociocultural background. Culture, ethnicity, and sociologic factors play an important role in the development of patterns of response to stress. Coping skills that are available to the individual when a crisis occurs may be largely a result of what has been modeled at home during times of crisis in childhood. It is difficult for American nurses to be cognizant of cultural norms of behavior for every culture represented in emergency patient populations, but in areas where a dominant ethnic group is heavily represented, it is helpful for nurses and physicians to learn about the cultural norms for individuals in the represented minority, including common responses during crisis and stress. It is understood, of course, that there are still great individual variations within any culture. Nurses should also identify the cultural influences that affect their own evaluation and judgment of patients. Racism and xenophobia can be poisonous influences disabling provision of unconditional care and treatment in EDs, and every effort should be made to eradicate these fear-based attitudes. Education and an open attitude toward the citizenry of the world now passing through EDs in every state can only benefit both health care providers and patients.

The fourth factor that influences the individual's response to crisis is spiritual background. Spirituality determines the way in which patients and significant others see themselves in relationship to other people, the way they view their purpose in life, and their relationship to the community and even the universe. Some people view accidents or illness as punishment from God for some known or unknown wrong or sin. Some people believe that God sends difficulties into their lives to help develop their character or to teach them a lesson. Many individuals belong to organized religions that guide them in their understanding about illness, injury, or tragedy. Representatives of organized religion may be a source of comfort or they may cause the patient or family agitation during a time of crisis. The patient or family may feel that the presence of a religious figure denotes impending death. The triage nurse's role in dealing with a patient's spirituality is not to form judgments about whether the individual has a reasonable belief but to ask the patient and/or significant others if the triage nurse may in some way facilitate their spiritual comfort. This may take the form of calling a priest, rabbi, or spiritual mentor, or it may take the form of allowing the patient space, quiet, and time to be alone with those who are a spiritual comfort to the individual.

It may seem paradoxic to assert that an unchanging element of triage is the individuals' response to tragedy while listing factors that affect that response, but the triage nurse's understanding of these factors is essential for quickly sizing up the situation she/he is presented with so that the patient receives individualized care. The triage nurse may also ponder the factors that affect an individual's response to stress in the face of tragedy to monitor his/her own makeup, while recognizing that our ability to provide unconditionally responsive care is affected by our own physical, psychologic, sociocultural, and spiritual well-being.

Many of us have been taught to avoid judging patients and families, but triage *is* a process of judgment. Triage personnel must make judgments about the individual's response to tragedy or an illness or accident that is a perceived threat in order to respond in a manner that is sensitive to the individual. Without a conceptual framework for understanding patients and others significant to them, triage personnel are at greater risk for responding in an insensitive and unprofessional manner or in a haphazard fashion that does not address the concerns of the individual. Triage nurses are also charged with continually deciding whom to triage first, and they must size up quickly who will be seen first in the triage area. Patients who are the most emotionally upset cannot always be seen first; this would be unfair and unsafe for those who have critical problems. If very emotionally upset individuals are seen immediately, it may be to evaluate the problem, offer comfort measures, and orient the individual to what will happen next, that is, tell them when they will be fully triaged.

PATIENT ORIENTATION TO TRIAGE AND THE EMERGENCY DEPARTMENT

Because most people entering an ED or health care facility for care are often fearful, it is always a good idea to orient them to the process of receiving care and to let them know who the individuals are that make up the health team. Patients' perceptions of the overall quality of ED care are enhanced when they are provided standardized information on arrival to the ED (Krishel and Baraff, 1993). Furthermore, patient compliance with therapeutic regimens is enhanced when standardized discharge instructions are provided in writing (Vukmir et al, 1993). Providing written orientation information and discharge instructions is a standard all EDs should enforce. It is particularly helpful, should patients return to the ED for a follow-up visit

---

CASE REPORT

A 29-year-old Caucasian woman, "Linda," brings her 9-month-old son to be seen by the ED physician. She is in tears as she tells the triage nurse that she has brought her son to be seen because he is "burning up" with fever. While the nurse takes vital signs on the baby, she intermittently interjects questions and comments about the child and family. She learns that although this is Linda's only son, she lost three older children in a tragic mobile home fire 2 years earlier. The nurse notices that Linda is grossly underweight, fatigued, and stressed. Her response to Linda includes recognition for the tragedy she has suffered in the death of her three older children while she affirms Linda's parenting of this child by praising her for seeking care for her child and for implementing appropriate fever-control measures at home. As time permits, the nurse requests a social work consult to discuss community counseling opportunities for Linda and offers Linda a glass of juice. The whole interaction between the triage nurse, patient, and parent takes no more than 5 minutes, but it is meaningful and helpful because the nurse has recognized Linda's individual response to her son's illness and has facilitated positive coping skills through beginning to address the factors that have an impact on Linda and her son's total family and physical health.

or reevaluation, since the triage nurse can pull the patient's chart and verify why the patient was seen and what instructions the patient was given on discharge.

It is an act of common courtesy for the triage nurse to introduce herself or himself as a registered nurse who will do a brief interview and assessment directly related to the patient's reason for seeking care. Patients should be informed that it is impossible for the triage nurse to predict the amount of time it will take for them to be seen in the ED or when they will even be brought back into the department for care. They should be informed regarding the principles of emergency care and triage: that the most seriously ill or injured are always evaluated and treated first. They should also be informed about the limitations of the triage nurse in providing treatment, and that simple first aid and diagnostic tests may be performed only as deemed immediately necessary. While the patient and family members are being oriented to the situation in the ED, it is important for them to feel that they have an advocate in the triage nurse and that he/she is approachable and concerned with their comfort and care. It should also be evident by the triage nurse's behavior that the waiting environment is maintained in as quiet and safe a condition as possible for the comfort of all.

The use of a volunteer or paid liaison in triage can be helpful in keeping the waiting area calm and sufficiently stocked with reading materials for health education and diversion. Liaisons are also helpful in maintaining communication between the ED staff and family, as well as between the triage nurse and patients (Sahnd, 1991). One research project studying patient satisfaction in the ED found that patients were more concerned with the caring attitude, communication skills, and organization of ED staff than they were with waiting times for ED service (Bursch et al., 1993). Another study conducted to evaluate patient perceptions of health care in the ED found that there was a direct correlation between the level of patient satisfaction with ED care and the amount of information the patient received at the time of arrival in the ED (Bjorvell and Stieg, 1991). ED staff should periodically seek feedback from patients about how the staff can communicate more helpfully, and patients should be informed of the mechanism for providing feedback about their care.

VARIATIONS IN ENVIRONMENT
Small Emergency Departments

The act of triage takes place in acute care settings in a variety of facility types. Perhaps the most challenging is not the level I trauma facility where resources are readily available but the small community facility where resources may not be readily available or accessible. Independent decision making is far more necessary in such a facility and has profound consequences for patient outcomes. In very small hospitals with EDs of fewer than 10 beds it is possible that only one or two registered nurses, a physician, and a medical assistant or emergency medical technician are employed. Although small hospitals may not have all the highly advanced technology or services of larger facilities, they often serve wide catchment areas and are faced with as great a variety of medical and injury presentations as large hospitals. Although the variety of problems brought to small EDs is similar to that in large hospitals, the frequency of high-acuity patients and the census level are less than at larger facilities, which means that nurses and physicians must persist in maintaining a high level of readiness and skills for nursing or medical assessments and care that may not be required often.

In small facilities it is important that the following issues be clearly addressed:

1. *Roles of personnel in triage and treatment should be clearly defined.* It is not uncommon in small facilities for the first patient interviewer to be a secretary or registration clerk. This condition is necessary because when there is only one registered nurse for an entire department, she/he may be busy doing a procedure or caring for a patient already in the department. When a registered nurse is not available to be the first interviewer for a patient requesting care, the second most appropriate person would be the medical assistant (MA) or emergency medical technician (EMT). That trained individual may be educated and supervised by the registered nurse in basic interviewing skills and may follow department policies for obtaining vital signs and clinical measurements and providing primary first aid until the registered nurse or physician is available

to do a more detailed assessment. Experienced MAs or EMTs are also astute at recognizing many emergent conditions such as myocardial infarction, airway obstruction, or burns that require immediate attention and care. When it is impossible for an adjunct medical person to interview patients arriving at the department, the secretary or registration clerk should be in a physical location that allows immediate access to the nurse to maximize patient safety. It is imperative that all department personnel are trained in cardiopulmonary resuscitation (CPR) and oriented to immediately alert the nurse when a patient has a problem that appears to threaten life or limb. All personnel who are first interviewers should be taught to introduce themselves by name and title to the patient to avoid confusion and inappropriate expectations.

2. *Principles of triage and assessment of acuity should be applied to patient care.* In small EDs, common sense is often relied on to dictate which patients receive care first. Levels of acuity are more often used for billing purposes than for care provision. Designation of acuity even in small hospitals can have advantages for objective service delivery and patient disposition. Nurses and physicians in small facilities should have a strong foundation in assessment of patients with traumatic injuries and use the preferred trauma scoring system for that facility or country. This procedure is important for prognostication as well as for triaging patients who qualify as ''trauma patients'' out to a trauma center if it would be to the patient's benefit. Ethical dilemmas can arise regarding triaging patients out, such as whether it is safe to transport the patient the distance required to reach a trauma center, the refusal of family members to have the patient transferred away from the area, and the possibility that a qualified surgeon (although not certified in trauma care) is more immediately available. Guidelines for coping with ethical dilemmas such as these are discussed in Chapter 13.

It is important for nurses in large hospitals who receive patients from smaller facilities to understand the working conditions of nurses in small community hospitals.

Small hospitals, particularly at night, have sparse staffing, and services such as pharmacy, laboratory, and radiology are frequently available only on an on-call basis. Limitations in the ready availability of laboratory data do not mean that clinical assessment skills are impaired; in fact, small-facility personnel often have highly attuned clinical diagnostic ability as a result of limitations in sophisticated laboratory and radiology adjuncts.

3. *Communication and interchange with area facilities are important.* Nurses and physicians from small facilities should avail themselves of opportunities to become oriented to triage policies and procedures in larger facilities, and vice versa. All health care facilities should work with community agencies such as the Red Cross to maintain a high level of disaster preparedness.

   Communicating the patterns of illness and injury seen in the patient population in small hospitals to area primary care providers and public health agencies is important. For example, when an outbreak of bacterial meningitis is encountered, notification of public health agencies is automatic, but a call to local school nurses to remind them about the signs and symptoms of the illness and to notify them of the problem is helpful in ensuring prompt recognition and treatment of any additional cases that may be seen in school health offices. Primary health care providers and occupational health care personnel also participate in preventive health care in educating their patients about ways in which infectious diseases and injuries can be avoided.

4. *Advocacy for consistently needed services should be persistent and documented.* Personnel in EDs of small facilities may lament the absence of certain laboratory tests that are not available for the diagnosis of their patients. Rather than passively accepting the limitations of the department and hospital's budget, when warranted, the hospital should conduct a cost-benefit analysis of obtaining needed testing equipment or services. Such a cost analysis should include the time required and cost of obtaining the test elsewhere, the potential damage to the public relations of the hospital

in patient dissatisfaction, and the potential for profit through making the service available.

5. *Use of ancillary personnel and family members is helpful.* In small EDs the ability to cope with a full or an over-flowing census is challenged. Prioritizing and delivering care can leave little time for patient teaching and commu-nication with families and patients regarding the status of the patient and what will happen next for that individual. It is wise at these times to enlist the support of ancillary staff such as hospital volunteers to expedite the triage and care process by assigning simple triage tasks such as ob-taining information regarding the patient's demographics for the registration process and recording why the patient is seeking treatment, what medications the patient is taking, and the presence of allergies to medication. A self-registration form may also be employed to allow the nurse or technician who triages the patient to quickly assess whether the patient has an emergent problem or can wait to be seen. Use of ancillary staff or a self-registration form speeds the triage and registration process and allows the patient to be oriented at an earlier stage to the process of triage and the status of the ED's census. This allows pa-tients an earlier courtesy option of obtaining care else-where, such as at an urgent care center, when they have a problem such as a simple laceration that can safely be treated at a nonacute care facility.

6. *Communication with the triage nurse or charge nurse in a larger facility to which a patient is being triaged out is important.* Nurses who "triage out" patients or who will accompany a patient on an interfacility transfer should first communicate with a charge nurse or triage nurse from the larger facility about the patient. A brief report including the patient's age, sex, chief complaint, vital signs, medi-cations, allergies, status at time of arrival, and current con-dition will be helpful in allowing the receiving nurse time to assign the patient to the appropriate area in the receiving ED. In addition, nurses at small facilities often have knowl-edge about the patient's family and support system that must be communicated to facilitate consideration of the

patient's comfort and needs when they arrive at the second facility. It is also helpful for the reporting nurse to include the current diagnoses the physician has established for the patient (realizing that the receiving hospital will reassess and diagnose the patient's condition independently when more diagnostic facilities are available). The reporting nurse need not apologize for limitations in diagnostic reports if they are not available because of lack of resources, but if, for example, the patient has not had radiologic evaluations and will not be bringing copies of films to the receiving hospital, the situation should be made clear.

7. *Transportation mode of patients "triaged out" of small clinics or hospitals to larger facilities should be safe and appropriate.* Nurses who are participating in triaging patients out of small facilities to larger hospitals must be familiar with county Emergency Medical Services (EMS) policies regarding patient transport. For example, an ambulance staffed with volunteers who are trained in CPR and first aid should not be used for a patient with an intravenous line and respiratory compromise unless absolutely necessary. If the patient is a critically ill pediatric patient, the outcome is more likely to be positive when a specialized pediatric transport ambulance team and ambulance facility are used (Johnson and Gonyea, 1993). If an advanced life support (ALS) ambulance is not available for a critically ill patient, it is appropriate for the nurse to request that a nurse or physician accompany the patient to the second facility. The benefits of rapid nonambulance transport versus waiting for ambulance transfer of a patient must be carefully but rapidly weighed when a deteriorating patient needs hospital ED care. In one study that evaluated the costs and benefits of transporting critically ill children to the ED, police transportation to the ED demonstrated shorter time to intubation for children with impending respiratory arrest; the authors concluded that nonambulance transport of critically ill pediatric patients should be considered in EMS policies (Sacchetti et al., 1992).

    If ambulance companies have safety policies regarding not transporting patients within a defined period after the patient receives medications, the nurse should have a baseline familiarity with these policies in order to give medications efficiently with consideration for the patient's impending transport. As in all situations, family members and others significant to the patient must be apprised of the impending transfer and should be oriented to the location of the receiving hospital so that transportation, if they wish to go to the receiving hospital, can be secured for them, particularly if the ambulance company does not allow family members to ride in the ambulance. The patient needs preparation and education regarding the transfer, to reduce fears when the transport team arrives.

Clinics and Schools

Like nurses and physicians in small hospitals, health care providers in clinics and schools are in a challenging situation for triage practice. Depending on the census and staff/patient ratios, health care providers in these situations can be overwhelmed at times by a rush of individuals needing service. Nonetheless, the same policies that govern triage in hospitals can be used to triage patients in clinics and schools. Ancillary staff such as student health aides or health clerks in the school setting may be used to obtain initial information from patients requesting services so that the patients can be triaged appropriately by the professional staff member. Ancillary staff should also be oriented to patient signs and symptoms that necessitate immediate notification of the nurse or physician to avoid disastrous patient outcomes (Box 2–2). Staff should also be trained in calming patients who are panicked about their situations. The ability to have a calm manner with patients is valuable in any health care delivery setting, and this is especially true with children who are frightened when ill or injured and not in the care of a parent or guardian whom they know and trust. Professional staff members are well advised to take a peek into the waiting area once in a while and get a quick look at the patients waiting to be seen to quickly identify any patients who appear very ill but may not have been deemed so by the ancillary interviewer. A brief look at the waiting list is also helpful in informing the

BOX 2–2	**Notification Guidelines for Ancillary Staff**

(When To Let the Nurse or Doctor Know That a Patient Has a Potentially Emergent Medical Need)

HISTORY COMPLAINTS

Difficulty breathing, foreign body aspiration, choking, loss of consciousness, seizure, chest pain, overdose, vaginal bleeding and pregnant, vaginal bleeding that soaks more than one pad per hour or in any patient who is pregnant, severe abdominal pain, vomiting blood, severe pain, fracture, possible neck injury, bee sting with history of allergy to bee stings, any significant medical problem with which the patient is experiencing a problem (e.g., diabetes).

PHYSICAL PRESENTATION

Unable to breathe and speak in sentences, audible wheezing, extreme pallor in face or injured limb, oral temperature higher than 101° F, tachycardia, orthostatic vital sign changes, extreme discomfort, loss of ability to walk or move an injured part including the neck, diaphoresis, disorientation or any change in normal mental status, seizure activity, laceration with uncontrolled bleeding, or severe injury such as near-amputation of finger

---

ancillary staff member of the probable triage order of patients and giving instruction and supervision for any simple care measures or assessments that may be helpful before the patient is formally seen by the professional. Ancillary staff can also be helpful in orienting patients to the process of triage and informing them about when they are likely to be seen. Ancillary staff can be efficient and helpful, but it is important to know their limitations in education and experience.

When a patient arrives at the clinic or school health office, the patient's health card or chart should be immediately accessed in order to determine whether the patient has a history of significant medical problems or allergies about which the professional should be apprised. Ancillary staff can be useful in notifying parents as needed and directed, but first a brief assessment of the patient by the professional is usually advisable, to avoid contacting family members unnecessarily. Use of 911 or emergency services when there appears to be a threat to life or limb should be instant to promote the best possible outcome for the patient. When emergency services that are not available in the clinic or school are needed for medical or legal reasons or to provide care not available on site but not immediately necessary, the facility should have a policy that is known by the staff regarding the use of ambulances staffed by emergency medical technicians or volunteer laypersons. Staff should never hesitate to use the 911 service when it is necessary for the safety of the patient, but overuse of emergency services for nonurgent problems is costly and wasteful. Whenever safe, it is preferable for the family to transport the patient for services. Again, guidelines and policies for "triaging out" patients by ALS and non-ALS ambulance or by the clinic or school care provider or family member in a private car should be developed by nurses and/or physicians and reviewed by legal experts. It is also useful for clinics and schools with patients who are frequent consumers of services, whether for necessary physical care or for emotional reassurance, to have their charts available so that the provider may review them for changes in status and problem identification and consider them for later discussion with primary health care providers.

It is important to recognize the differences between triage in small hospitals and clinics and in larger hospitals so that the limitations and strengths of small facilities are clear to those providing care in larger facilities. Likewise, the triage process and services of a larger facility must be understood by personnel in small facilities so that they can prepare patients and family members for the experience they may have when being sent to a large facility. Having a dual picture of emergency services also allows for a greater sense of collegiality, as well as criticism because misunderstanding is avoided.

Field Care Situations

Patients who are triaged from "the field" for care in acute care facilities are often evaluated under chaotic circumstances that make it difficult to obtain an accurate, complete assessment of the history and presentation of the individual. Field personnel are usually trained in the ABCDE (mnemonic) method of assessment: the patient's *a*irway, *b*reathing, *c*irculation and *ce*rvical spine, and *d*isability from injuries or illness are systematically evaluated through obtaining vital signs and *e*xposing the patient in order to fully observe injuries. Other mnemonics and brief assessment tools specific to the patient's chief complaint are used, such as the CMTS (*c*irculation, *m*otor, *t*emperature, and *s*ensation) mnemonic, which is used for checking the neurovascular integrity of an injured extremity. These assessment tools are discussed in Chapters 8 and 9. They are mentioned here to remind all triage personnel that there are methods for rapid and accurate field assessment, and it is important for both the reporting and the receiving professional to obtain all pertinent information from the time of the patient's earliest assessment. Ensuring consistent transmission of information from the field assessment is helpful in reevaluating the appropriateness of the patient's triage at the hospital and then in tracking changes in the patient's condition from the field.

It is valuable for nurses and personnel in EDs to take periodic ambulance rides as observers in order to more fully understand the assessment process and the conditions under which field personnel perform their assessments. In addition, it is helpful for the field personnel: hospital professionals sometimes have good suggestions for improving field assessment and care.

Large Hospitals With Trauma Units

Triage in hospitals with large trauma units is perhaps the most straightforward situation in which triage is performed. Assigned roles and responsibilities of department personnel are well defined, and the consistent use of objective criteria to designate the acuity level of patients in triage and on direct arrival into the department by ambulance is ensured by frequent quality assurance studies.

Services such as radiology, laboratory, and pharmacy are also readily available, as well as assessment adjuncts such as pulse oximetry—all of which, as discussed earlier, are not always available in smaller hospitals, clinics, or schools. Despite the advantages of triaging patients in a large hospital with a trauma system, wide variations in the physical location of triage, the role of the triage nurse, and the policies that govern triage exist.

In some facilities the triage nurse is also the charge nurse. This means that the triage nurse must not only assess incoming patients and designate their acuity level but also determine where patients are to be seen in the ED, communicate with family members and significant others, and deal with ED issues such as patient admissions to the units within the hospital, incoming ambulance patients, and personnel issues such as staff breaks. The disadvantage of this situation is that the nurse assigned to triage and charge has myriad responsibilities, and the sensory overload from a number of different sources can be constant. The advantage to this arrangement is that the triage/charge nurse has more direct responsibility for the time frame in which patients will be seen and the power to move patients into the department if they need to be seen immediately. Access to the physician is direct because the triage/charge nurse is not usually responsible for direct patient care in the ED.

In some hospitals the triage nurse is assigned solely to the triage area. This situation allows the triage nurse to direct her/his full attention to the assessment, triage care, and acuity designation of patients and to give attention to the periodic reassessment of patients who must wait in the waiting area before being brought back to the ED.

A disadvantage of this arrangement is that the triage nurse must depend on the charge nurse's cooperation and must trust her/his triage acuity assessments and trust her/him to bring patients into the ED in a timely, fair manner. If the triage nurse is physically separated from the interior of the ED and patients in the waiting area have to wait long periods to be seen, the triage nurse may be on the ''firing line,'' with angry, uncomfortable patients who direct their frustration and unhappiness to the only representative of the ED directly available to them—the triage nurse. In EDs where security risks are a great concern, that is, every ED without a metal detector and police officer, the triage nurse can be an unprotected ''sitting duck'' for any patient who is at risk for violent behavior. In this situation the triage nurse should have immediate access to the security department and full encouragement to use the 911 service to access police services if necessary for her/his personal safety or the safety of patients in the triage and waiting areas.

One disadvantage of having a nurse assigned solely to

triage is the potential cost-inefficiency of this role during slow periods. When a triage nurse is located within the ED, it may be possible for that person to help with brief procedures and care of patients in the ED. Some EDs try to make the triage role cost-efficient by assigning the triage nurse to make "call-backs" whereby patients who have been seen in the ED recently are telephoned to evaluate their comfort and compliance. This act of courtesy can be misinterpreted as insincere, however, if the triage nurse must cut the call short to care for an incoming patient. An argument for not having the triage nurse participate in ED patient care or call-backs is the unpredictability of patients arriving in the parking lot or triage area with immediate needs, such as the emergent labor and delivery patient, cardiac or respiratory arrest patient, or drive-up trauma patient.

The safety, working comfort, and cost-efficiency of the triage nurse should be a consideration for new EDs debating the physical location of a triage area and whether it will be housed within the front of the ED or separate from the ED. Determining whether triage will be a singular role or combined with another responsibility such as charge nurse should involve the input of ED personnel and involve discussions with personnel of other area health care facilities about their experiences with triage issues and practice.

Perhaps one of the greatest challenges faced by triage nurses in a large facility is the high volume of patients during peak service hours. For some EDs this is a 24-hour situation. In EDs where nurses work 12-hour shifts, it is important to ensure that the triage nurse, as well as all nurses in the department, get regular breaks. Rotating the triage nurse's assignments after 4 or 6 hours is also advisable, to provide variation in job stimulation and the opportunity for a number of nurses in the ED to maintain proficient triage skills. Triage nurses should be communicated with on a regular basis by the management of the ED to obtain the nurses' impressions of the patterns of patient presentations, patient satisfaction, and quality care issues so that system-specific problems in the delivery of care can be addressed and ways to prevent frequent illnesses and injuries with the help of the public and occupational, school, and primary health care professionals can be identified. In an effort to maintain a smooth-flowing triage area, it is helpful for triage nurses to have ancillary staff available for translation, communication with family members, assistance with simple first aid such as applying ice packs to sprains, and as in smaller hospitals, clinics, and schools, obtaining basic demographic and medical information that can then be validated.

No matter what the setting for triage is, it should be performed in a systematic, efficient, and kind manner. Nurses should maintain a high level of education regarding acuity designation policies and should communicate whenever necessary and helpful with their colleagues in other facilities involved in care of patients arriving at the ED for treatment.

REFERENCES

Adamowski K et al: Sudden unexpected death in the emergency department: caring for the survivors, *Can Med Assoc J* 149(10):1445, 1993.

Bjorvell H, Stieg J: Patients' perception of the health care received in an emergency department, *Ann Emerg Med* 20(7):734, 1991.

Bursch B, Beezy J, Shaw R: Emergency department satisfaction: what matters most? *Ann Emerg Med* 22(3):386, 1993.

Cooke MW, Cooke HM, Glucksman EE: Management of sudden bereavement in the accident and emergency department, *Br Med J* 304(6836):1207, 1992.

Gagnon L: Customer service: is the answer better communication? *J Emerg Nurs* 17(2):63, 1991.

Johnson CM, Gonyea MT: Transport of the critically ill child, *Mayo Clin Proc* 68(10):982, 1993.

Krishel SM, Baraff LJ: Effect of emergency department information on patient satisfaction, *Ann Emerg Med* 22(3):568, 1993.

Sacchetti A, Carraccio C, Feder M: Pediatric EMS transport: are we treating children in a system designed for adults only? *Pediatr Emerg Care* 8(1):4, 1992.

Sahnd S: Making the ED waiting game a little easier to play, *RN* 54(1):19, 1991.

Thomas D: How to deal with children in the emergency department, *J Emerg Nurs* 17(1):49, 1991.

Vukmir R et al: Compliance with emergency department referral: the effect of computerized discharge instructions, *Ann Emerg Med* 22(5):819, 1993.

Walters D, Tupin J: Family grief in the emergency department, *Emerg Med Clin North Am* 9(1):189, 1991.

RECOMMENDED READING

Heiskell LE, Pasnau RO: Psychological reaction to hospitalization and illness in the emergency department, *Emerg Med Clin North Am* 9(1):207, 1991.

Jackson LE: Understanding, eliciting, and negotiating clients' multicultural health beliefs, *Nurs Pract* 18(4):30–32, 37–39, 42, 1993.

Johnson CM, Gonyea MT: Transport of the critically ill child, *Mayo Clin Proc* 68(10):982, 1993.

Kanter RK et al: Excess morbidity associated with interhospital transport, *Pediatrics* 90(6):893, 1992.

Walters D, Tupin J: Family grief in the emergency department, *Emerg Med Clin North Am* 9(1):189, 1991.

3 Triage in Disaster Situations

DISASTER MANAGEMENT

"Triage in disaster situations" brings the concept of triage full circle, back to its origins. Sorting wounded soldiers into treatment categories is as old as war itself, and war is the worst of all disasters since it is initiated and perpetuated by human beings. Triage procedures continue to be followed by armed services departments in overseas military actions such as the Persian Gulf War. Although conditions in war are unique, the priority of triage—identifying individuals requiring emergent care first and transporting them to a place where assessment and stabilization can occur—does not differ in disasters outside of war (Burkle et al., 1994). American hospitals and field personnel have not been called to act in triage scenarios relevant to war on American soil since the Civil War. Triage as it relates to disasters in America is now a process that occurs during natural disasters such as the floods in the summer of 1993 in the Midwest, Hurricane Andrew in Florida in 1992, and the San Francisco Bay area earthquake of 1990. These large, devastating disasters involved rescue efforts in the field, as well as exhaustive efforts on the part of hospital personnel to meet the many needs of a community.

Smaller-scale events qualify as disasters when they challenge the ability of a staffed acute care facility beyond its resources. A bus accident involving multiple injured passengers may be considered a disaster, as may a building that collapses and injures many people. Local events that produce multiple injured patients are particularly devastating in rural areas that have limited acute care facilities to handle patients triaged for care to emergency departments (EDs). The ideal situation following a disastrous event is when patients are successfully triaged to many acute care facilities in such a way that no one

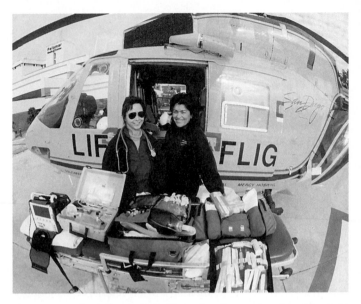

Fig. 3–1   A high level of readiness for disaster is critical for field care and acute care.

facility is overtaxed and the necessity of a "disaster" code is avoided.

What is considered a disaster then must be defined by both field conditions and acute care facility conditions and readiness (Fig. 3–1). Furthermore, although acute care facilities may easily be able to provide care to patients who have survived or been injured in a disastrous event, the designation of "disaster" status to an emergency event is necessary for purposes of economic assistance and to ensure readiness of acute care personnel to handle anticipated emergency patients.

DISASTER READINESS

Disaster readiness is the key to handling a disaster efficiently and with minimal mortality and morbidity. Disasters generally requiring a high degree of readiness are listed in Box 3–1.

Disaster readiness in general can be elicited through avail-

| BOX 3–1 | **Disasters Requiring Specific Readiness** |

- Airline accidents
- Avalanches
- Bombs
- Chemical explosions
- Earthquakes
- Floods
- Hazardous material accidents
- Hurricanes
- Nuclear or radiation disaster
- Tornadoes

---

ability of physical supplies, designation of staff for various duties in the event of a disaster, rehearsal of disaster drills in which personnel enact their designated roles in a "mock disaster," and cooperation of community and acute care hospital facilities in communicating their policies and procedures in the event of a disaster. Specific disaster readiness is also necessary in areas where specific types of disasters are high risks. When policies are revised for field care personnel and acute care facility workers, the experiences of others in disaster situation care should be considered.

In the 1989 Loma Prieta earthquake, 63 people were killed and 3700 were reported injured; the services of 51 hospitals were required, and there was a 15% increase in ED census (Pointer et al., 1992). Minor trauma was the most common complaint, although there was, in the more injured or ill, a slight increase in the rate of hospitalization. Although the emergency services were busy but not stressed, difficulties identified in handling this disaster included problems with disaster intelligence, communications, emergency medical services (EMS) dispatch, obtaining patient care records, inadequate disaster training, and hospital damage (Haynes et al., 1992). In many disaster critiques and reviews, organization and communication are emphasized again and again. Use of a command post, with everyone knowing her/his job and performing it almost in a rote fashion, is thought to be the greatest guarantee for efficiency, particularly since "mechanical actions override processes requiring thinking and judgment" during times of disaster (Johnson and Gamble, 1991).

To deliver the best care to all patients, consideration for special populations is necessary. In the Avianca Flight 52 crash of January 25, 1990, 22 of the 25 children aboard this jet survived. Problems occurring in the rescue of all surviving passengers included excessive responders (three ambulances per patient) and confusion (a near-crash of two helicopters after the crash) (Dulcharsky et al., 1993). Specific problems identified in the care of the surviving children were related to inadequate triage and transportation for optimal care, as well as inadequate pediatric training of responding personnel and deficiencies of the regional plan in considering the needs for pediatric designations (van-Amerongen et al., 1993). Use of scoring systems have been identified as helpful when triaging trauma victims following a disaster, as in the case of the Kegworth M1 airplane crash (Rowles et al., 1992). Disaster planning should build on the systems and tools of triage and emergency care but should be inclusive and consider specific disasters, which types of patients may be involved and their special needs, and community and personnel resources.

Safety of personnel is a primary factor that facilities and personnel must consider when planning disaster readiness and actions. Individuals working in emergency situations are often expected to behave in heroic ways that endanger their own personal safety. Although this may be morally laudable, it is not practically efficient. Workers who endanger themselves and are injured or killed are no longer available to provide critically needed care for others. As personnel are trained in disaster readiness, the concept of considering the good of "the whole" should be imbued in order to prevent unnecessary loss of personnel during disaster rescues and care. With this approach it is possible for personnel to give themselves permission to avoid dangerous situations that may compromise their safety and ability to provide care for others. Disaster readiness means that personnel should also be able to be self-sufficient for at least the first 72 hours following a disaster with their own food and water (Alson et al., 1993). Appropriate clothing and medical gear are also critical, particularly if triage and rescue personnel are working in harsh weather conditions (Johnson and Gamble, 1991) or at risk of contracting lethal infections, as did the firefighter who contracted "toxic strep" (*Streptococcus pyogenes*) from a child on whom he performed cardiopulmonary resuscitation (CPR) (Valenzuela et al., 1991).

Physical Readiness

Physical readiness for disasters includes the perpetual maintenance of emergency equipment in optimal condition. In field care agencies maintenance of rescue equipment is imperative. Stocking sufficient supplies relevant to specific anticipated disasters is critical for both field care and acute care agencies, as well as designated community care facilities that may need to respond during disasters to local patient needs. In areas where earthquakes are a high risk, all agencies need to follow American Red Cross guidelines for stocking survival supplies and be concerned with the potential for communication problems and physical isolation in case access roads, bridges, and telephone lines are destroyed. It is important that management personnel keep abreast of what survival and emergency care supplies are available in order to communicate with triage personnel in apportioning therapeutics during triage. This will ensure that supplies are efficiently used. For example, after a devastating earthquake, patients triaged for care will have a variety of problems: crush injuries, isolated head injuries, and stress-induced medical crises such as myocardial infarctions and asthmatic crises, as well as the normal patient flow of individuals with tubal pregnancies, acute surgical conditions, and so on. When a hospital is isolated and has limited supplies, those who triage and direct initial care may need to be conservative in determining which patients are monitored and which patients receive intravenous therapy, more so than in nondisaster situations when supplies are not rationed. Triage personnel need to immediately ask themselves, "Is this treatment necessary to the continuance of life or limb?" and "What is the likelihood of survival of this individual even in the case of aggressive and immediate treatment?" There is no time for ethical dilemmas during a disaster; when there are limited supplies and multiple patients, the most critical patients with the highest likelihood of survival are given the most aggressive therapy. Furthermore, the authority of the triage team in the field must be absolute, since they have firsthand knowledge of the scope, magnitude, and details of the situation (Klein and Weigelt, 1991).

Specific supplies that should be available in all disasters (Box 3–2) include management and respiratory support equipment for respiratory failure, circulation support equipment (intravenous therapy supplies) for hypovolemia, medication for pain management and treatment of airway disease, and basic supplies such as blankets and water. Any method of recording patient information—clearly who they are, their designated level of acuity, and what their chief complaints, vital signs, and allergies are—is appropriate and helpful to those in acute care receiving facilities. Marker pens or sticker labels can be used. It is not helpful to recommend computer-generated forms for patients, since computers may not function during a disaster. It would also be helpful to record other information such as current medications, but it is unlikely that there will be sufficient time, and only if the individual is critically dependent on medication (e.g., insulin) should triage personnel take the time to record medication. Using a permanent-style marker that is clearly visible on the patient is more helpful because it will

---

BOX 3–2	**Basic Disaster Equipment**

- Airway resuscitation equipment
- Blankets
- Cellular telephones
- Insulin
- Intravenous therapy equipment
- Labels or tags
- Oral and nasopharyngeal airways
- Oxygen
- Permanent markers
- Tetanus toxoid
- Trauma scissors
- Water

not get lost and will ensure that the information is instantly available to receiving personnel. Toe tags are cumbersome to tie and may get lost, and they have a frightening association for patients who realize that toe tags are usually used only when patients are headed for the morgue.

Physical readiness in disaster situations involves knowing what to do with "extras" who arrive at a disaster scene or facility to assist with care but who are not hired by the agency responsible for triaging or receiving and caring for patients. Although many managers with legal concerns would advocate a brief, courteous "thanks but no thanks" response consideration of how to best use or direct volunteers should depend on the size of the disaster and how well personnel are managing without additional assistance.

Although personnel may be handling the physical aspects of the job, victims of disaster are often in psychogenic shock or are frightened or upset and need the comfort and presence of professionals educated in providing psychologic support.

Psychologic Readiness

Psychologic readiness, like physical readiness, is best ensured through the systematic preparation of personnel who may provide care in disaster situations. The following information is provided personnel: their roles and responsibilities in a disaster (such as triage, radio, field care, acute care, and medical duties), the physical layout of the triage and emergency adjunct areas, and who they are responsible to in a disaster situation. Personnel need to be encouraged to take care of their own physical needs during prolonged hours of a disaster in order to maintain the ability to think clearly and provide excellent care. Mental health professionals included in a disaster team should be informed about the possible consequences of specific disasters so that they may anticipate the psychologic effects on patients and care providers. Since many patients seek care for minor health concerns because of anxiety, the goals of psychologic intervention are to reinforce effective functioning and encourage complete functioning as soon as possible so that overcrowding of health care facilities is prevented. Mental health professionals can also encourage health care providers who are giving physical care to victims of disaster and can communicate with family members of those affected by disaster (Rosenbaum, 1993). Reassurance and compassion are simple but essential ingredients in the care given to patients during disaster and in the treatment of team members by one another during high-stress times (Pepe and Kuetan, 1991).

Designation of volunteers to bring care providers water and food is invaluable to preserving the mental and emotional capabilities of disaster personnel providing direct patient care.

FIELD CARE

On arrival at a disaster scene, personnel should already be aware of their specific duties (Box 3–3). The overriding concern of all personnel, however, as directed by their team captain, should be assessing the environment for safety hazards and determining the safety of the environment as a working area. If the area is determined to be unsafe as a working area, a determination of when, how, and by whom rescue operations will take place is made before the triage of patients begins. A physical area to which patients will be rescued must be determined and cleared. If the physical area where patients are found is determined to be safe, triage evaluations can be initiated and initial basic life

---

BOX 3–3	**Triage in Disaster Field Care**

- Assess the physical safety of the area.
- Designate and clear an area for care if present area is unsafe.
- Visually sort patients into categories of immobile wounded, walking wounded, and noninjured.
- Number patients clearly (with a marker).
- Assess all patients and potential patients for triage designation according to presentation acuity (airway compromise, CRAMS scale score, mechanism of injury, and vital signs).
- Record critical information on patients as they are assessed: name, chief complaint, vital signs, allergies, and critical information (e.g., diabetic).
- Triage patients out according to designated acuity level and viability.

---

support (BLS) and advanced life support (ALS) care instituted. All patients who have been up and walking since the disaster occurred should be encouraged to sit or lie down pending an evaluation. Those who were immobilized by injuries should not be moved until they have been assessed. The triage person designates numbers to the patients (1, 2, and so forth) for easy communication to receiving facilities. Acuity designation is then determined based on the patient's presentation (obvious signs of acute distress), CRAMS score (see Chapter 1, Box 1–12), mechanism of injury, and vital signs. Chief complaint and allergies should also be noted for the benefit of those in acute care receiving facilities but do not affect acuity designation unless directly related to the patient's condition. Patients with critical medical problems and those who will require maintenance medications relevant to their conditions should be noted and the information also clearly marked on the patient's hand or body tag as time permits.

Every effort should be made to work quietly and efficiently to maintain an optimal psychologic environment for patients and minimize their stress. Excessive stress increases the potential for mortality and morbidity. Individuals who are not critically injured and who are mobile, and the "walking wounded" who are highly emotional (i.e., who are screaming or crying), should be separated if possible from those with critical injuries to promote a better working environment and reduce the stress level on critical patients who may be frightened by the situation. Personnel must also monitor their own affect and communication style in order to maintain a calm demeanor, thereby reassuring patients.

In prolonged rescues or if sufficient emergency transport vehicles are not available to transport patients for acute care, a second triage phase must be instituted. During this phase the ABCDEs of emergency patient assessment and care (the mnemonic is presented in Box 3–4) are more fully instituted; if patients have already received a full ABCDE evaluation, treatment based on deficits in these areas may be instituted as equipment permits.

Patients awaiting transportation should be kept calm, quiet, and warm, and should have frequent reassessment of vital signs and overall status. When acuity changes necessitate that a patient designation be changed, the change in status should be

BOX 3–4	Disaster Evaluation and Care Based on ABCDE Mnemonic

AIRWAY

Evaluate airway patency
Institute oral or nasopharyngeal airway as necessary
Provide suctioning as necessary

BREATHING

Evaluate for obvious signs of distress (e.g., stridor)
Evaluate respiratory rate, rhythm, and depth
Evaluate chest for bilateral breath sounds and expansion
Evaluate for clinical signs of hypoxia (e.g., pallor, cyanosis)
Instruct the patient to breathe as normally as possible
Encourage relaxation and a focus on calming thoughts

CIRCULATION AND CERVICAL SPINE

Evaluate pulse and blood pressure
Evaluate for neck and back pain
Initiate intravenous therapy if indicated
Initiate cervical spine precautions if indicated
Monitor dysrhythmias or indicate if cardiac complaint or history

DISABILITY

Evaluate for fractures
Evaluate neurovascular status of injured extremities
Align and secure injured extremities

EXPOSE

Expose the patient by cutting off clothing and assessing for injuries
not obvious on initial presentation
Do systematic assessment for system-specific injuries and treat in
order of life-threatening status

---

made and communicated to receiving facilities. When transport
is prolonged, treatment should continue with particular effort to
reduce trauma-related morbidity such as infection (e.g., clean
and bandage wounds if not already done) and hypothermia (e.g.,
keep patient warm and dry).

ACUTE FACILITY CARE

Patients who enter an acute care facility from a disaster situation where they have been triaged are reevaluated and retriaged according to presentation and level of acuity on arrival (Fig. 3–2). To determine the appropriate designation, triage personnel in acute care must consider the report of the field personnel, the patient's presentation on arrival, the CRAMS score and vital signs, and further information that may be rapidly obtained in an acute care setting, such as oximetry and "quick-look" monitor evaluations. In acute care facilities triage is directed by physicians and nurses working within a framework understood by both. Triage personnel in acute care facilities often provide orders, as well as designate staff to provide care, and it is important that these be clear, written if possible, and appropriate to the patient. As at the disaster scene itself, when multiple

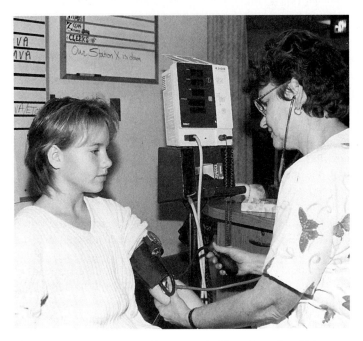

Fig. 3–2 Reassessment of an acutely ill patient should be performed periodically during the waiting period in the emergency department.

patients are involved, predesignated areas must exist for receiving incoming patients. Additional personnel responding to assist in a disaster should be directed to areas appropriate to their specialties. As mentioned earlier, appropriation of services in the case of multiple patients and highly acute conditions is determined by the availability of services and the viability of patients. Such decisions are made by triage personnel and the medical director of emergency services in the facility receiving patients.

Throughout the assessment and treatment phases of care for disaster victims, personnel should be sensitive to the need of family members to receive communication about their loved ones. Ancillary personnel are used for communicating with family members of patients when possible, giving family members clear instructions on whether they may come into the treatment area or, if not, when they will be allowed to see the patient. Reassurance of both patient and family members is an important factor in minimizing the effects of stress on the patient's physical and psychologic health. When at all possible, patients should be allowed to see and be comforted by family members, however briefly, as long as family members are able to maintain a calm demeanor and are able to encourage the patient. It is the right of individuals to receive love and comfort from their families during times of crisis. If the patient is not likely to survive, it is appropriate to seek the services of support personnel who are trained chaplains, psychotherapists, or social workers to stay with the individual and the family until the patient dies. This act recognizes the human dignity of the patient and the need for comfort at the time of death.

Disasters are not only *treated* in acute care facilities; they can *occur* in acute care facilities. Because a hospital may be directly affected by natural and human-made disasters, hospitals must maintain updated policies and procedures for responding to internal disasters; the following topics should be addressed: loss of power; loss of water; destruction of an area by fire, flood, or bomb; staffing issues; evacuation; and communication with outside agencies (Aghababian et al., 1994). Triage during internal disasters may be a slow process if structural damage occurs. For example, the Musgrave Park Hospital bombing in Belfast, November 1991, involved the slow extrication of pa-

Table 3–1 Triage Considerations for Specific Disasters

Disaster	Common patient problems	Triage considerations
Earthquake	Crush injuries	Careful evaluation of abdomen and chest
	Isolated head injuries	Careful assessment of neurologic status
		Periodic evaluation for increasing intracranial pressure (ICP)
Flood	Drowning	Appropriate care for near-drowning victim (i.e., airway support, warm blankets, assessment for fluid and electrolyte imbalance)
	Infectious disease	Evaluation for signs of infection (gastrointestinal and respiratory)
		Careful history regarding exposure to contaminated water and/or food
Nuclear disaster	Nuclear fallout	Protection of personnel from nuclear contamination
		Treatment of individual for nuclear contamination before entering acute care facility
		Psychologic response of victim
Chemical explosion	Airway compromise	Investigation of specific contents of chemicals involved and communication with appropriate agency (e.g., poison control center) to discover immediate hazards from exposure for personnel entering area as well as patients affected by explosion
		Frequent assessment of airway patency and oxygenation

Continued.

Table 3–1 Triage Considerations for Specific Disasters—
cont'd

Disaster	Common patient problems	Triage considerations
		Immediate delivery of oxygen in the case of potential or actual respiratory compromise
		Observation for immediate and refractory smoke or chemical inhalation signs and symptoms and appropriate treatment
		Decontamination
	Burns	Assessment of damage to critical anatomy and estimated body surface burned and thickness of burns
		Triage to burn care center whenever possible
		Concurrent intravenous access and fluid replacement during triage process
		Appropriate treatment according to specific criteria for specified chemical
Tornado	Crush injuries	Careful evaluation of abdomen and chest
	Isolated head injuries	Careful assessment of neurologic status
		Periodic evaluation for increasing intracranial pressure
	Lacerations	Assessment for arterial bleeding and damage to critical organs such as eyes
		Concurrent bandaging as appropriate to degree and location of laceration
Hurricane	See Tornado, Flood	

Table 3–1 Triage Considerations for Specific Disasters—
cont'd

Disaster	Common patient problems	Triage considerations
Airline accident	Smoke inhalation	Assessment of respiratory status and support of airway and breathing
	Burns	Assessment of damage to critical anatomy and estimated body surface burned and thickness of burns
		Triage to burn care center whenever possible
		Concurrent intravenous access and fluid replacement during triage process
	Psychologic trauma	Assessment of whether patient has lost friends or family in accident
		Enlistment of support personnel
Avalanche	Suffocation	Assessment and support of airway and breathing
	Crush injuries	Careful evaluation of head, spine, chest, and abdomen
	Hypothermia	Assessment and maintenance of core temperature
		Assessment for dysrhythmias
		Assessment of extremities for neurovascular status

tients through a narrow portal access (Hodgetts, 1993). The only advantage of this situation is the ability to set up conditions helpful for dealing with the dead and optimizing the survival of the injured.

Further information on how to be prepared for disasters is available from the American Red Cross. Common injuries, illnesses, and triage considerations for specific types of disasters are summarized in Table 3–1. The information in Table 3–1 is not all-encompassing, but acute care facilities can draw from the information to develop their own disaster readiness and in-servicing for disaster response.

As mentioned earlier, the experience of individuals who have provided triage and care services in disaster situations should be sought in order to learn from their mistakes and strengths when maintaining and updating plans for disaster response in both field care and acute care. One hospital, which has managed two commercial airline crashes and one military helicopter crash, realistically reported that when real disasters with high numbers of dead and injured patients are involved, the best that can be hoped for is "controlled chaos" (Klein and Weigelt, 1991). Confusion, problems with communication, and determining who was in charge improved with each successive disaster, but these problems affirmed the need for an organized, systematic, even rigid approach to triage roles, responsibilities, and hierarchy for efficient care.

MOTOR VEHICLE DISASTER SITUATIONS

Although *disaster* most commonly refers to accidents of nature or those involving unusual circumstances such as a building collapse or an airline accident, a motor vehicle accident that involves many vehicles or patients may also be deemed a disaster when the need for services and care overwhelms the agencies that are typically well prepared to handle fewer critically ill or injured patients.

Safety considerations for personnel who work at motor vehicle accident scenes must be foremost. Attention to cordoning off a safety zone is imperative in the earliest phase of emergency response. Accidents involving one or two vehicles can become multiple-vehicle accidents if other drivers pay more attention to the accident than to their driving. Cooperation of the highway patrol in managing traffic at the scene of an accident is invaluable.

Field considerations specific to motor vehicle accidents involve gaining a rapid understanding of the nature of the accident, determining the physics of damage to vehicles with inferred understanding of the implications for patient consequences, and questioning what appears to be obvious for missing pieces of information. The accident is evaluated by learning the speed of the vehicle(s) involved, how and what the vehicle(s) struck at any points of impact, and whether the vehicle(s) rolled over. The physics of damage to vehicles is evaluated with particular attention to passenger space intrusion (from any direction) and the potential hazard of fire or explosion.

Inference about patient consequences based on vehicle damage includes consideration of what part of the patient's body impacted the vehicle interior or was affected by forces of acceleration or deceleration. In addition, conditions specific to the interior of the vehicle must be considered (e.g., whether the patient was restrained and, if so, with what type of restraint, and whether flying objects or unrestrained passengers may have collided with other passengers who were restrained). "Questioning the obvious for missing pieces" includes consideration of the potential for missing persons as a result of ejection from the vehicle or persons being hidden in wreckage from the accident. Rescue workers and field care providers need to be astute in noticing clues such as an unoccupied carseat, reports of patients verbalizing concern over a missing person, and evidence of missing persons at the scene such as a trail of blood not associated with a patient found at the scene.

Field triage is similar to enactment of triage in any disaster. One difference, however, is in the event of deaths of patients involved in a motor vehicle accident. Death of a passenger automatically raises the index of suspicion for triage and treatment personnel that others involved in the accident may qualify for designation as trauma patients. In addition, although disasters such as earthquakes, with many injured and dead persons, may require that the deceased be merely covered while treatment and triage of the living continue, clearing an accident of deceased victims is necessary for the psychologic safety of other patients involved. This scenario is more likely in a motor vehicle disaster than in a devastating earthquake. A word of caution, however: patients who are thought to be "dead" should in fact be *carefully assessed* to verify this condition. Pulselessness and apnea should be verified by physical assessment and through cardiac monitoring.

ENACTMENT OF TRIAGE FOR MULTIPLE PATIENTS WITH MEDICAL ILLNESS

Evaluating patients in disasters with the primary consequence of medical illness requires that triage personnel use their assessment skills astutely and with great accuracy. Patients with injuries are more easily sorted into acuity levels based on the threat that their injuries pose to life or limb. Patients with medical illness require evaluation of their level of compromise and of the likelihood of their condition worsening.

Smoke Inhalation

Inhalation injuries can be organized into three types: acute asphyxia, in which the victim is usually dead at the scene; upper airway heat damage, which causes progressive airway edema and obstruction; and small airway damage that is manifested early (2 to 5 days) as adult respiratory distress syndrome (ARDS) or late (after the first week) by bronchopneumonia (Purdue and Hunt, 1991). Not only victims of fire but also firefighters who may be in close and continued contact with smoke may have smoke inhalation. Because the body initially adapts, the patient with smoke inhalation may at first experience only a cough and nausea. However, decompensation results in an acute respiratory condition with reduced likelihood of survival. Individuals who triage patients in a setting where smoke inhalation has been experienced by a number of patients must first remove all patients from the immediate area if possible. The demand of the patient's body for oxygen must then be reduced by placing the patient in a sitting or supine position. Finally, triage into acuity levels is performed based on the presence of obvious airway compromise as evinced by the patient's respiratory status (respiratory rate, rhythm, and depth and movement of air on auscultation) and signs of inadequate oxygenation such as pallor or cyanosis. Maintaining as calm an environment as possible is also necessary to minimize the stress and oxygen demands on the patients. Meeting their other physical needs, for example, providing a warm blanket, is also helpful and comforting. Triage personnel must also be prepared to evaluate the condition of rescue providers who may experience smoke inhalation due to the duration and nature of their contact with smoke.

Principles that apply to triaging multiple patients with smoke inhalation also apply to triaging individuals with chemical exposure that causes respiratory compromise. Triage personnel should assist rescue personnel managers in ensuring that providers wear appropriate respiratory equipment during exposure to smoke or airborne chemicals.

Hypothermia

Hypothermia, which may produce medical illness, may occur in an avalanche, when victims are trapped in snow, in near-drowning or with prolonged exposure to cold water as in boating accidents, or with exposure in the wilderness, when an individual becomes lost in a cold climate. Triaging hypothermic patients requires recognition that, to minimize loss of extremities, treatment must be concurrent with assessment. Depending on how cold victims are, attention should first be paid to assessing and maintaining the core body temperature, evaluating the metabolic effects of hypothermia, particularly on the cardiac system (assess for dysrhythmias and hypotension), and initiating core warming as early as possible. Patients with the worst neurologic and cardiac signs of hypothermia should be triaged as emergent. Patients should then be triaged according to the stability of their condition at the time of evaluation and the likelihood of complications and deterioration as judged by their age, overall health status, and preexisting medical problems. Specific actions taken to meet the needs of the hypothermic patient include removing the patient from the cold, removing wet clothes, applying a warm blanket, avoiding moving the patient excessively, and protecting frostbitten parts. In the triage assessment, another ''D''—for *d*egree of temperature—should be added to the ABCDE evaluation of the patient if possible, particularly on arrival at a care facility (Britt et al., 1991).

Infections

Steinberg and Nichols (1991) hypothesized that there is always an increased risk of infection following tornadoes, hurricanes, and mass trauma situations because of infection barrier disruption resulting from injury, changes in living conditions, and disruption in usual medical care, as well as factors specific to the disaster itself. Tornadoes, hurricanes, and volcanoes, for example, cause an increased release of dirt into the atmosphere, resulting in the release of *Clostridium perfringens* into the air, thereby increasing the likelihood of gas gangrene, particularly in high-risk patients such as those who are immunocompromised. Although deaths from natural disasters such as tornadoes have been reduced in the last 20 years because of improvement in early-warning systems (Centers for Disease Control, 1994), postdisaster consequences cannot be totally eradicated. Triage professionals should be apprised of community risks for an increase in specific infectious diseases so that they may watch for signs and symptoms of these infections. Minimizing the risk of infection following a disaster may be addressed as indicated in Box 3–5.

Morbidity was minimized as a result of the excellent triage, assessment, and care that occurred following the Andover, Kansas, tornado of April 26, 1991. There were 22 deaths and many injuries. The injuries were primarily of soft tissue with foreign body contamination, as well as many fractures. The low complication rate from these injuries, which normally carry a high risk for infection, was attributed to thorough and early open-wound management (Rosenfeld et al., 1994). A low incidence of infection in patients with open wounds following a terrorist bomb blast in Victoria Station, London, in 1991 was also attributed to early surgical wound debridement (Johnstone et al., 1993). This type of success begins with appropriate triage and triage care of injured patients. Not all disaster reviews have

---

BOX 3–5	**Minimizing the Risk of Infection Following a Disaster**

- Management of the dead through efficient removal and safe disposition of the bodies
- Management of waste and sewage
- Prevention of vermin and insect reproduction
- Provision of adequate shelter
- Mass immunization for those who are not immunized or are underimmunized

reported such a positive outcome. After the Mt. Pinatubo volcanic eruption there were 349 deaths in the first 12 weeks, largely because inadequate water, waste disposal, and shelter caused outbreaks of measles, acute respiratory infections, and diarrhea (Surmieda et al., 1992). Following the 1985 volcanic eruption in Armero, Colombia, the fourth largest volcanic cataclysm in the history of humankind, there were more than 23,000 deaths and 4500 wounded. Many of the victims suffered from necrotizing fasciitis and mucormycosis, early recognition and treatment of which are essential if death from infection is to be prevented (Patino et al., 1991). The January 1994 earthquake in Northridge, California, left 170 persons in Ventura County with a diagnosis of acute coccidioidomycosis between January 24 and March 5 (as compared with 52 cases in all of 1993). This increase in the incidence of coccidioidomycosis was probably related to increased release of airborne dust. The incubation period of this disease, 1 to 4 weeks, coincided with the earliest reported cases following the earthquake (Centers for Disease Control and Prevention, 1994a). As stated previously, consideration of the potential infectious agents released into the air is important, as is the early availability of basic medical services.

Hurricane Iniki, which occurred on September 11, 1992, left 614 patients with hurricane-related health concerns; most sought care for primary health problems and all were treated successfully with basic medical services and primary health care (Henderson et al., 1994). Likewise, reports published after Hurricane Andrew (August 1992) indicated that most of the care provided was routine medical care; depletion of tetanus toxoid, antibiotics, and insulin supplies occurred within 24 hours of the disaster (Alson et al., 1993), and no outbreaks of enteric or respiratory disease were reported among the high population of armed service members in the area (Lee et al., 1993). It was reported that disease outbreaks were prevented by relatively rapid restoration of utilities, sanitation, and primary health care availability (Hlady et al., 1994). Following Hurricane Hugo in September 1989, one of the most frequent complaints of the 2090 treated patients was insect stings; 26% of these patients had general reactions to the stings (Brewer et al., 1994). More than just germs are stirred up in the environment following a windy disaster, and triage personnel must be prepared to evaluate individuals suffering insect stings for anaphylaxis and other general medical crises, as well as injuries.

Concerns regarding risk of infectious disease following a disaster should be uppermost in the minds of rescuers regarding their own health as well as the health of the people they care for. This is true in American disasters and even more so for disasters in developing countries, to which volunteers from around the world respond with relief efforts and crisis intervention.

The most profound, ongoing global disaster at this time is the displacement of persons from their homes, primarily as a result of civil strife and war. In 1990 there were 300 million displaced persons in the world; there are more than 43 million today. The death rate in this population is greatest in children younger than 5 years of age, and in all groups deaths occur most often as a result of diarrhea, measles, and respiratory infections, which have devastating effects on individuals who are immunocompromised as a result of chronic malnutrition and inadequate water, sanitation, and shelter (Toole and Waldman, 1993). In the 1988 Bangladesh floods, the worst floods in the history of that country, 46,740 patients were treated and 154 deaths were reported, most frequently caused (in all patients younger than age 45 who died) by diarrhea (Siddique et al., 1991). The causes of death in displaced persons are most often preventable or treatable with the proper implementation of public health standards and basic medical care such as immunization and administration of fluid therapy and antibiotics. However, to be effective in helping others, as already mentioned, rescuers must protect themselves against infection by having adequate vaccination and maintaining good health (Aghababian and Teuscher, 1992).

When approaching a disaster, triage personnel must identify the specific risks of infection, isolate and treat infected patients, and prevent the spread of infection. This process should be ongoing throughout the following phases of a disaster: *impact* (0 to 4 days), when extrication and initial treatment are taking place; *post-impact* (4 days to 4 weeks), when airborne, foodborne, and waterborne infections may begin and the number of endemic infections may increase, even to epidemic proportions; and *recovery* (after 4 weeks), when infections with

Table 3–2 Triage Concerns for Infectious Disease During a Disaster

Time frame	Concerns	Actions
Impact phase (0 to 4 days)	Protection against tetanus and other vaccine-preventable diseases such as measles	Evaluate wounds for early signs of infection. Consider risk factors for infectious diseases (water and sanitation) and engage in preventive teaching.
Post-impact phase (4 days to 4 weeks)	Airborne (e.g., coccidioidomycosis), foodborne (e.g., salmonella), and waterborne infections	Review the nature of endemic infections (e.g., malaria) and evaluate patients for these.
Recovery phase (after 4 weeks)	Infections with a long incubation period	

a long incubation period may become evident (Aghababian and Teuscher, 1992). Specific clinical concerns relevant to the phases of disaster are summarized in Table 3–2.

Triage history questions should focus on the exposure of the patient to a disaster, the current living situation and conditions, and compliance with public health recommendations for sanitation, potable water, and food. Sometimes patients with infectious disease are not in a disaster-stricken area but have traveled from that area; thus there is value in asking all patients in whom infection is suspected whether and from where they have traveled in the weeks prior to seeking health care.

In the 1993 Midwest flood, 524 flood-related conditions in patients were reported; 47.7% were injuries and 44.5% were illnesses. The health problems of the public were primarily related to population displacement and disruption of normal health services during the initial phase (July 15 to September 3, 1993) (Centers for Disease Control and Prevention, 1993), but concerns about mosquito-borne disease continued long after the flood was over because of stagnant waters and CDC reports of 200 mosquito bites per hour (Cotton, 1993). Triage and health personnel must be familiar with vector-borne infections such as malaria, dengue fever, and encephalitis, particularly if such an infection has been reported in a disaster-stricken area.

Exposure to Hazardous Material

Approximately 2000 of the 60,000 chemicals produced in the United States are considered hazardous materials by the Department of Transportation. Disasters involving hazardous materials must be anticipated in areas where these chemicals are transported, pass through, or are in use. Triage personnel need ready access to information regarding specific hazardous materials and their medical consequences. Teamwork between physicians and all ancillary personnel is critical in this type of crisis for determining the implementation of a disaster plan and the treatment of exposed patients. Personnel must be attired properly for work in an area where a hazardous material accident has occurred.

The triage interview of patients exposed to hazardous material includes questions about the chemical or chemicals to which they have been exposed, the length and duration of exposure, and the surface area exposed. During the interview, if not already done, the patient should be stripped of contaminated clothing and provided with materials for washing with soapy water in a decontaminating area (unless contraindicated). Physical assessment should include determination of any injuries and initial therapy that has been instituted. Care and concern for critical structures such as the eyes should be foremost in the minds of triage personnel, and inspection of warm, moist areas such as the groin and axillae, which rapidly absorb chemicals, is recommended (Leonard, 1993). Secondary contamination of a treatment area during decontamination should be prevented by designation of a ''hot zone'' or decontamination area specific for patient reception and decontamination (Kirk et al., 1994).

Chemical gas clouds can be highly lethal and may necessitate rapid evacuation of an area involved in such a disaster. Chlorine is the chemical most commonly implicated in gas cloud accidents, and it is critical for triage personnel to evaluate the respiratory status of patients affected by chlorine gas exposure, since rapid death resulting from bronchospasm or edema, or both, of the respiratory structures is possible (Baxter, 1991).

Minor burns caused by caustic chemicals should not be dismissed as nonurgent, since systemic toxicity may ensue as a result of exposure to a lethal chemical via the skin (Cooke and Ferner, 1993). Therefore all chemical burns resulting in severe pain and discomfort should be triaged as emergent. Irrigation of exposed skin should also be immediate unless contraindicated (Shibata et al., 1994).

Exposure to Radiation

Accidental irradiation may occur in either a therapeutic or an industrial environment. The exact mechanism of injury is not well understood, but the effects of acute radiation injury are known to have consequences in the skin, gastrointestinal tract, bone marrow, and gonads (Hirsch and Bowers, 1992). In the beginning of the triage process the patient must be evaluated for the presence of traumatic injuries (blunt, penetrating, or burn) as well as irradiation, since these patients must receive immediate medical intervention. The patient must be questioned about the type of radiation exposure, proximity to the source, duration of contact, and any decontamination procedures used. Policies and procedures for decontaminating the patient according to county and agency standards must be followed. Simply removing the victim's clothing and bathing the skin with soap and water are sufficient for decontamination in 90% to 95% of cases (Hirsch and Bowers, 1992). Health care providers are not considered at risk for radiation contamination in caring for the vast majority of victims of irradiation, although assurance of personnel safety is not possible until decontamination of the patient is complete.

SUMMARY

Victims of disasters of any type who are trapped for prolonged periods without their basic needs being met are at risk for dehydration, infection, exhaustion, hypoxia if the air supply has been compromised, psychologic crisis, and complications related to preexisting medical conditions that require routine therapeutics or medication. Furthermore, these patients may also have traumatic injuries that have gone untreated when they were not accessible to rescue personnel.

Assessment of such individuals should be brief and based on ABCs of basic life support, and therapies essential to maintaining life instituted while transporting the patient as quickly as possible for acute care assessment and therapy. Acute care triage of these patients must involve family members who may be able to comfort and encourage patients to fight for survival. The psychologic well-being of a patient who has been traumatized for a prolonged period is paramount for physical stabilization.

Triage of patients in disaster situations requires that triage personnel take time to appraise the situation, consider the physical safety of the area for personnel and patients, designate treatment personnel, and use the principles of triage methodically and swiftly in an effort to save lives and limbs. Excellent care during times of disaster requires that both field and acute care facility personnel are always ready for disasters, in particular, those for which their region is at high risk. Emergency personnel should be encouraged to participate in local disaster relief agencies to maintain up-to-date knowledge of disaster preparedness and an understanding of how their skills can be most helpful in the event of a disaster. Emergency personnel also have a community responsibility to model disaster readiness in homes and be prepared to provide education in their community schools and support organizations.

REFERENCES

Aghababian RV, Teuscher J: Infectious diseases following major disasters, *Ann Emerg Med* 21(4):362, 1992.

Aghababian R et al: Disasters within hospitals, *Ann Emerg Med* 23(4):771, 1994.

Alson R et al: Analysis of medical treatment at a field hospital following Hurricane Andrew, 1992, *Ann Emerg Med* 22(11):1721, 1993.

Baxter PJ: Major chemical disasters, *Br Med J* 302(6768):61, 1991.

Brewer RD, Morris PD, Cole TB: Hurricane-related emergency department visits in an inland area: an analysis of the public health impact of Hurricane Hugo in North Carolina, *Ann Emerg Med* 23(4):731, 1994.

Britt D, Dascombe W, Rodriguez A: New horizons in management of hypothermia and frostbite injury, *Surg Clin North Am* 7(2):345, 1991.

Burkle FM Jr, Orebaugh S, Barendse BR: Emergency medicine in the Persian Gulf War. Part I. Preparations for triage and combat casualty care, *Ann Emerg Med* 23(4):742, 1994.

Centers for Disease Control and Prevention: Morbidity surveillance following the midwest flood—Missouri, 1993, *JAMA* 270(18):2164, 1993.

Centers for Disease Control and Prevention: Coccidioidomycosis following the Northridge earthquake—California, 1994, *JAMA* 217(22):1735, 1994a.

Centers for Disease Control and Prevention: International decade for natural disaster reduction, *JAMA* 271(23):1822, 1994b.

Cooke MW, Ferner RE: Chemical burns causing systemic toxicity, *Arch Emerg Med* 10(4):368, 1993.

Cotton P: Health threat from mosquitoes rises as flood of the century finally recedes, *JAMA* 270(6):685, 1993.

Dulchavsky SA, Geller ER, Iorio DA: Analysis of injuries following the crash of Avianca Flight 52, *J Trauma* 34(2):282, 1993.

Haynes BE et al: Medical response to catastrophic events: California's planning and the Loma Prieta earthquake, *Ann Emerg Med* 21(94):368, 1992.

Henderson AK et al: Disaster medical assistance teams: providing health care to a community struck by Hurricane Iniki, *Ann Emerg Med* 23(4):723, 1994.

Hirsch EF, Bowers GJ: Irradiated trauma victims: the impact of ionizing radiation on surgical considerations following a nuclear mishap, *World J Surg* 16(5):918, 1992.

Hlady WG et al: Use of a modified cluster sampling method to perform rapid needs assessment after Hurricane Andrew, *Ann Emerg Med* 23(4):719, 1994

Hodgetis TJ: Lessons from the Musgrave Park Hospital bombing, *Injury* 24(4):219, 1993.

Johnson DE, Gamble WB: Trauma in the arctic: an incident report, *J Trauma* 31(10):1340, 1991.

Johnstone DJ et al: The Victoria bomb: a report from the Westminster Hospital, *Injury* 24(1):5, 1993.

Kirk MA, Cisek J, Rose SR: Emergency department response to hazardous materials incidents, *Emerg Med Clin North Am* 12(2):461, 1994.

Klein JS, Weigelt JA: Disaster management, lessons learned, *Surg Clin North Am* 71(2):257, 1991.

Lee LE et al: Active morbidity surveillance after Hurricane Andrew—Florida, 1992, *JAMA* 270(5):591, 1993.

Leonard RB: Hazardous materials accidents: initial scene assessment and patient care, *Aviat Space Environ Med* 64(6):546, 1993.

Levin DL et al: Drowning and near-drowning, *Pediatr Clin North Am* 40(2):321, 1993.

Patino JF et al: Necrotizing soft tissue lesions after a volcanic cataclysm, *World J Surg* 15(2):240, 1991.

Pepe PE, Kvetan V: Field management and critical care in mass disasters, *Crit Care Clin* 7(20):401, 1991.

Pointer JE et al: The 1989 Loma Prieta earthquake: impact on hospital patient care, *Ann Emerg Med* 21(10):1228, 1992.

Purdue G, Hunt J: Inhalation injuries and burns in the inner city, *Surg Clin North Am* 2(2):385, 1991.

Rosenbaum C: Chemical warfare: disaster preparation in an Israeli hospital, *Soc Work Health Care* 18(3–5):137, 1993.

Rosenfield AL, McQueen DA, Lucas GL: Orthopedic injuries from the Andover, Kansas, tornado, *J Trauma* 36(5):676, 1994.

Rowles JM et al: The use of injury scoring in the evaluation of the Kegworth M1 aircrash, *J Trauma* 32(4):441, 1992.

Schnitzer PG, Bender TR: Surveillance of traumatic occupational fatalities in Alaska—implications for prevention, *Public Health Rep* 107(1):70, 1992.

Sheehy S, Jimmerson C: *Manual of clinical trauma care,* ed 2, St Louis, 1994, Mosby.

Shibata K, Yoshita Y, Matsumoto H: Extensive chemical burns from toluene, *Am J Emerg Med* 12(3):353, 1994.

Siddique AK et al: 1988 floods in Bangladesh: pattern of illness and causes of death, *J Diarrhoeal Dis Res* 9(4):310, 1991.

Steinberg SM, Nichols RL: Infections and sepsis in disasters, *Crit Care Clin* 7(2):437, 1991.

Surmieda MR et al: Surveillance in evacuation camps after the eruption of Mt. Pinatubo, Philippines, (published in erratum appears in *MMWR-CDC Surveill Summ* 41[51]:963, 1992); *MMWR-CDC Surveill Summ* 41(4):9, 1992.

Toole MJ, Waldman RJ: Refugees and displaced persons. War, hunger, and public health, *JAMA* 270(5):600, 1993.

Valenzuela TD et al: Transmission of 'toxic strep' syndrome from an infected child to a firefighter during CPR, *Ann Emerg Med* 20(1):90, 1991.

van-Amerongen RH et al: The Avianca plane crash: an emergency medical system's response to pediatric survivors of the disaster, *Pediatrics* 92(1):105, 1993.

RECOMMENDED READING

Borak J, Sidell FR: Agents of chemical warfare: sulfur mustard, *Ann Emerg Med* 21(3):303, 1992.

Grieshop TJ, Yarbrough D III, Farrar W: Case report: phaeohyphomycosis due to *Curvularia lunata* involving skin and subcutaneous tissue after an explosion at a chemical plant, *Am J Med Sci* 305(6):387, 1993.

Hallagan LF, Smith M: Profound atelectasis following alkaline corrosive airway injury, *J Emerg Med* 12(1):23, 1994.

Michaelson M: Crush injury and crush syndrome, *World J Surg* 116(5):899, 1992.

Pepe PE, Kvetan V: Field management and critical care in mass disaster, *Crit Care Clin* 7(20):401, 1991.

Stewart CE: *Environmental emergencies,* Philadelphia, 1990, Williams and Wilkins.

4 | Cultural Considerations

LANGUAGE BARRIERS TO HEALTH CARE

The primary mechanism for triaging patients is the patient interview. If the triage professional is unable to interview a patient because of a language or communication barrier, it is important to resolve this problem as efficiently as possible. Every patient should initially be addressed in English to determine the patient's ability to comprehend and speak English (Diaz-Gilbert, 1993). The assessment of the patient's comprehension should be based on appropriate verbal responses rather than nodding, since patients may at first be reluctant to reveal that they do not speak English. If the patient's primary language is not English, the triage professional should access a translator as soon as possible to gain a clear understanding of the patient's chief complaint and symptoms and to obtain any information necessary for appropriate triage (e.g., the presence of allergies or medications) (Fig. 4–1).

One commonly used method for accessing translators is for a facility to maintain a list of personnel working within the agency who speak languages other than English. This list should also indicate when personnel are available. If the individual who will translate arrives in the triage area, the nurse should determine the translator's ability to speak and understand English. Triage and other health care professionals who use nonmedical translators need to use lay terminology to increase understanding.

Translators who are not professionally trained for this role may be timid about asking the health care professional to explain medical terminology. Despite the translator's effort to be helpful, if she/he does not understand what the professional wants to know, the translator may not ask the appropriate questions.

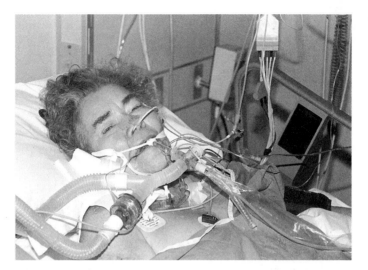

Fig. 4–1   Although this Asian-American female patient does not fit the profile of a heart attack victim, (white male over age 40), she suffered a myocardial infarction nonetheless. Triage assessment must not be bound by stereotypes.

Out of necessity and for expedience, children of non–English-speaking patients are frequently called on to translate. The drawback of this approach is that the child's ability to comprehend English and translate accurately into the native language may be limited. Patients with complaints they find embarrassing to their child may withhold crucial information regarding their chief complaint. Concerns and valuable information that the patient would like to discuss with the health care provider may then be omitted. If children must be used to translate, the health care professional should have children recite back in English what they understand they are to translate. This practice will help reduce inaccurate translation and instructions to the patient (Haffner, 1992).

A national service that provides translators by telephone who can ask the necessary questions and provide information in English to the English-speaking professional is used by many health care facilities (Box 4–1). This service is particularly

| BOX 4–1 | **AT&T Language Line Services** |

1 (800) 752–6096

Translation available 24 hours a day, 7 days a week for more than 140 languages

---

useful for patients who speak a language for which there is no hospital translator or when dialects are unfamiliar to translators. It is available for a nominal fee.

The optimal method for dealing with language barriers is to have a translator available specifically in the emergency department (ED), particularly when there is a high population of non–English-speaking patients. Professionally trained translators are an advantage to health care providers not only because of their ability to translate medical terminology but also because they usually have a highly developed level of cultural literacy. For example, when asked about the number of pregnancies they have had, Mexican patients will often report the number of pregnancies resulting in live births, not counting miscarriages or therapeutic abortions—a misunderstanding most easily revealed by a professional translator (Haffner, 1992). Patients with little experience in American health care, such as refugees or immigrants, are more likely to access care if they know that translators are available in a health care facility, since their primary concern is that their health care provider understand their problems (D'Avanzo, 1992).

Translators working in an ED are usually trained to take medical histories, but unless they are licensed health care professionals, they should not be expected to direct the interview based on the patient's presentation and responses to history questions. Translators are often cross-trained and able to provide other services within the department. They may act as translators for physicians providing patient care and during discharge teaching as well.

One method of working with non–English-speaking patients in triage is to use a printed triage questionnaire that is available in a variety of languages. This method allows the triage professional to access the information rapidly and to communicate in a number of languages. Written discharge instructions have been demonstrated to improve communication with ED patients (Isaacman et al., 1992), although some studies have shown a high proportion of illiteracy among randomly evaluated ED patients (Jolly et al., 1993). One obstacle to using translated written interview materials is that they require literacy of the patient. They also require use of multiple-choice or ''yes/no'' responses, since it is unlikely that the triage professional can interpret longer answers. Furthermore, using multiple-choice or ''yes/no'' responses on a questionnaire limits the details and subtleties elicited during an interactive interview. If translated triage forms are used by a facility, the triage nurse should make an attempt to identify the most literate individual in the family and to communicate primarily with that individual (Morgan, 1993). Another problem with this method is that it may not be practical when patients seek medical attention with severe pain or other symptoms that make it untenable for them to complete a questionnaire. When possible, this method can be used as an adjunct when translators are available, since it will shorten the time that the translator needs to interview the patient. This factor is especially critical when translators who work in other capacities within the hospital are used, since they may not be able to spend extended periods away from their primary responsibilities. Use of voice-generated translation— 40 commands that are available in over a dozen languages— during fluoroscopy has been reported to be successful, as demonstrated by the patient's ability to correctly follow the command given by the technician (Cohn and Cohen, 1994).

One language barrier that may become evident in triage is the patient who is deaf or unable to speak in a manner that can be easily understood, such as a patient with global cerebral palsy. The first task of the professional is to establish which method of communication the patient typically uses—signing, writing, or using a teletype system. Once the professional has established with the patient the easiest method of communicating, it is appropriate to ask the patient how the professional can best receive the information. Unless the patient is critically ill or injured, it is possible to await a response. When a non-verbal patient is critically ill or injured, the patient must be triaged on the basis of presentation and physical assessment. An effort should be made to obtain critical information through secondary sources such as Medic Alert bracelets, written records accompanying the patient, or family or others significant to the patient. Since it may be especially frightening for deaf patients to receive care in critical situations when they cannot hear or participate in decision making, every effort should be made to access a sign language interpreter, perhaps a family member or friend of the patient. Professionals living within areas with a high population of deaf or hearing-impaired persons would be wise to learn signs most often used in health care situations, such as the signs for pain and medicine. Pencil and paper should be available at all times for deaf individuals, and they should be clearly instructed on how to request help if they require assistance for any reason. If a central desk receives all patient calls, a note should be attached to the phone system to alert desk personnel that a deaf patient's call light must be answered in person.

Health care providers should remember that patients who do not speak English or who cannot speak are not helped by having the provider speak loudly at them. While it may be helpful for the professional to communicate slowly and clearly, the words selected should be spoken at the same volume that is appropriate for any other patient with a similar developmental and education level.

When a patient has a language or communication barrier or if the patient speaks English but it is not her/his primary language, the nurse should document the information. The nurse should also document what primary language the patient speaks.

It is often frightening for patients with communication barriers to access health care and to be triaged for their problem in such a way that they do not feel that their needs are clearly understood. Although the professional may not always be able to access translation or communication assistance in as timely a manner as would be ideal, it is important to convey to the patient that such methods are being sought. Comforting measures that are culturally appropriate should be used, such as a reassuring touch on the arm or a smile and sympathetic look. Touch must be used in a culturally sensitive manner, since touch may be perceived as a bonding, positive action or as an intrusive act (Giger and Davidhizar, 1995), depending on the culture.

Professionals performing triage who take into consideration how a patient with a communication barrier feels are truly providing care centered on the whole person. They are establishing a positive relationship between the patient and the health care provider, which improves the likelihood of patient compliance with recommended therapeutics in the treatment phase of care.

CULTURAL BARRIERS TO HEALTH CARE

Many immigrants now living in this country come from areas in the world where health care and the economic conditions are very different. The experiences and conditions of immigrants before their arrival in the United States are often responsible for chronic health problems and general health status (Uba, 1992). For example, physical trauma, malnutrition, and inadequate shelter are commonly reported in the health histories of immigrants from Southeast Asia, Russia, and South and Central America. Alternatively, immigrants who at one time enjoyed professional status and economic stability based on their position and government subsidy in their own country may be disoriented after arriving in America, where they may not be able to work as professionals and may be relegated to a low socioeconomic status.

Prior experience with health care systems in an immigrant's home country makes it difficult for the patient to understand how to access and use the health care system in the United States. Expectations may be unrealistic if patients believe that all things, including miracles, are not only possible but routine in the United States. Patients coming from countries where health care is not readily available usually appreciate the relatively easy access to health care in the United States and often associate good care with being treated kindly (Brod and Heurtin-Roberts, 1992). Only a health care professional who is willing to take a few extra moments to learn where the patient is from and ask about his or her previous experiences with health care in the country of origin will gain significant information about how the patient's life history may affect her/his health care and health perceptions. Triage nurses should ask patients what they believe caused their illness, as well as what benefit they hope for in accessing health care (Grossman, 1994). Including questions such as these during the triage process enlightens the nurse about the patient's cultural beliefs related to health and how these beliefs may affect patient care in the ED, not only for patients new to the United States but for all patients, since it cannot be assumed that a patient does not have cultural biases. Many black Americans, for example, equate health problems with bad luck, chance, fate, poverty, domestic turmoil, or failure of home remedies (Giger et al., 1992). Even individuals with many years of education may have personal beliefs that conflict with a traditional biomedical view of disease. Health care providers must not impose their beliefs on patients but must work within each patient's framework whenever possible in developing a relationship and providing information.

If immigrants are not educated regarding the appropriate use of the ED and how to access routine health care, overuse of the ED may become a problem. Public education (in a variety of languages) about the existence of and access to community health clinics and primary health providers is crucial in preventing this problem.

HOME REMEDIES AND FOLK MEDICINES

When patients are initially interviewed in triage, whether in a field care situation or health care agency, they are usually asked about medications they may be taking—both over-the-counter medications and prescription drugs. A vital omission can be made when patients are not asked about the use of home remedies. Many home remedies and folk medicines are simple and harmless and do have beneficial psychologic or physical effects. Some home remedies, however, can be harmful when used in excess or incorrectly. Severe exogenous lipoid pneumonia was reported in one patient who took many capsules of squalene (derived from shark liver oil and readily available in most Asian markets) for persistent hiccups before and during hospitalization for pneumonia (Asnis et al., 1993). Even substances that may appear harmless, such as garlic, have been reported to have serious consequences when used in a deleterious fashion; for example, a 6-month-old baby had second-degree burns after topical rubbing of the wrists with garlic (Garty, 1993). Because of the lack of quality control and safely regulations, infectious diseases resulting from the use of contaminated folk medicines have also been reported (Hufnagel and Schein, 1992).

Patients who arrive at triage with unusual or vague symptoms should be questioned carefully and patiently about the use of home remedies. A patient who has used a home remedy should be asked to provide a sample if possible. Samples of home remedies may be used for chemical analysis if necessary for an accurate patient diagnosis. The Chinese herbal medicine hai ge fen has caused lead poisoning (Markowitz et al., 1994), which was verified by means of chemical analysis. Arsenic and mercury intoxication has also been reported from the use of East Indian ethnic remedies (Kew et al., 1993). ''Herbal'' remedies may also contain prescription medications that can be harmful to patients; for example, one patient took herbal tablets that were produced in Mexico and were found to contain triamcinolone, which caused glucocorticoid excess and proximal muscle weakness (Capobianco et al., 1993). Ethnic or home remedies may be derived from a misunderstanding about how the remedy was used in the home country or a revival of a home remedy that had not been used for a long time. For example, chemical pneumonitis was reported in one child of Turkish origin whose parents used wool dipped in kerosene to relieve mild upper airway congestion, but the remedy resulted in pulmonary irritation, pneumonia, and dermatitis (Nussinovitch et al., 1992).

Home remedies are not exclusive to foreign-born patients but are also traditional and passed down from generation to generation in many families and are endemic to certain regions. Patients with terminal diseases may use herbal remedies, vitamins, or folk medicines in an effort to prolong life and optimize their quality of life. In one study of 114 patients with human immunodeficiency virus (HIV), 22% of the patients reported using one or more than one herbal product in the prior 3-month period, some in toxic doses with deleterious consequences (Kassler et al., 1991). As with religious and spiritual belief systems, when professionals have well-developed knowledge, at least about home remedies that are frequently used in the region where they practice or among populations known to use non-traditional therapies, they will be astute at questioning patients about their use of home remedies. Patients might at first be reluctant to provide information to health care providers in acute care settings, but they are more likely to trust providers who have knowledge of home remedies and who can ask about them specifically, by name.

In addition to considering the use of home remedies that are ingested, health care providers need to be familiar with home remedies that are applied, such as poultices. Furthermore, folk practices that are not common to conventional Western medicine must also be considered during the triage process. Otitis externa and facial cellulitis caused by the use of Japanese *mimi kaki* or Korean *kwi shi shi gee,* instruments made of bamboo with a carved-out spoon at one end, have been reported. The potential for infections resulting from the use of these instruments is significant, since 6000 to 7200 of these instruments are sold annually to the Japanese community in southern California alone (Berry and Collymore, 1993). Coin rubbing is a practice used by some Vietnamese patients and other Southeast Asians whereby a copper coin or another metallic coin is rubbed vigorously on the affected area from which the patient's symptoms are thought to originate. The friction this practice requires is quite rigorous, and it is common for the patient on whom coin rubbing is performed to have marked erythema or ecchymoses. A provider who is not knowledgeable about this practice or who has not inquired about the use of home remedies or ethnic health practices might mistakenly assume that the patient has been intentionally physically abused. Overzealous coin rubbing can be dangerous. One patient had an intracerebellar hemorrhage after a painful 30-minute ''coining'' (Ponder and Lehman, 1994). Cupping is another practice common among Southeast Asians whereby a small cup is heated and placed on the skin; negative pressure during cooling results in circular ecchymoses. Also common is moxibustion, which involves making small, round burns on the skin with incense or another instrument for this purpose (Buchwald et al., 1992). Another practice, in which fine scratches are made over a prescribed area, has been reported in Mien patients whose origins are Laotian (Gilman et al., 1992).

Examiners must be careful in communicating the need for information regarding the use of home remedies and folk practices. It is common for people to use or do things at home that they find beneficial, and these may include things that are not commonly prescribed by health care practitioners but that patients like to use to help themselves heal or feel better. Professionals must be nonjudgmental while indicating that they are genuinely interested in learning the information. Home remedies, although commonly herbal, may interact with prescribed medications or medications used in emergency situations. Therefore it is helpful to know ahead of time exactly what the patient has used at home.

Home remedies that are often used in the Hispanic population indigenous to Mexico, California, and South America are listed in Table 4–1. Most of the listed remedies have been in use since the time of the Aztec Indians, who developed not only a pharmacologic listing of herbs and substances used for healing but their own empirical chart and pharmacopeia. Some of the remedies may have originated in China. It is not unusual for individuals who use home remedies to also access Chinese herbal remedies such as ginseng and practices such as acupuncture. When examiners discover that practices such as acupuncture have been in use, it is helpful to know who performed the acupuncture and whether sterilization of the acupuncture needles was guaranteed (as is the case when it is performed by a licensed practitioner).

During the triage and interview process the examiner considers the patient's chief complaint, his/her use of home remedies and practices, and his/her rationale for such use.

If the triage professional is concerned about the possibility of an overdose of a home remedy, the poison control center should be contacted for further information and direction. Furthermore, it is important to encourage the patient to share information regarding overdosage of the particular substance with others who might also be at risk, and it may be helpful for emergency professionals to also make a referral to the public health department.

SPIRITUAL COMFORT: MOMENTS THAT COUNT

Consideration of the patient's spiritual needs during emergency care often depends on the provider's personal sensitivity to spirituality and his/her own belief system. If a provider does

Table 4–1   Some Common Mexican and Hispanic Folk
Remedies (Remedios Caseros)

Spanish	English
Manzanilla	**Chamomile**
Té: Dolor de estómago, cólicos menstruales, resfriados, migraña, cólicos.	*Tea:* Stomach pain, menstruation cramps, cold, flu, migraines, colic
Compresas de té: Hemmorroides, fístulas, ulceras, inflamación ocular	*Tea-soaked compresses:* Hemorrhoids, fistulas, ulcers, eye inflammation
Hierbabuena (té)	**Mint (tea)**
Dolor de estómago, flatulencia	Stomach ache, flatulence
Canela (té)	**Cinnamon (tea)**
Digestión, flatulencia	Digestion, flatulence
Ruda (té)	**Rue (tea)**
Sedante nervioso, histreria, dolor de estómago, naúseas	Nerve sedative, nervous prostration, hysteria, stomach ache, nausea
Ruda con chocolate	**Rue with chocolate**
Produce contracciones uterinas, migraña	Produces uterine contractions, migraines
Oregano (té)	**Oregano (tea)**
Insomnio, nerviosismo, ansiedad, broncodilatador, fiebre del heno	Insomnia, nervousness, anxiety, bronchodilator, hay fever
Cebolla morada (jarabe)	**Red onion (syrup)**
Tos ferina	Whooping cough
Ajo	**Garlic**
Reumatismo, picadura de insectos	Rheumatism, insect bites and stings

Table 4–1 Some Common Mexican and Hispanic Folk Remedies (Remedios Caseros)—cont'd

Spanish	English
Tila (té)	**Linden blossom (tea)**
Sedante nervioso, jaqueca	Nerve tranquilizer, sedative, sick headache
Belladona (tintura)	**Belladona (tincture)**
Mal de San Vito, epilepsia, hemmorroides, fisuras del ano	Epilepsy, hemorrhoids, anal fissures
Naranjo (té)	**Orange (tea)**
Sedante nervioso	Tranquilizer
Limón	**Lemon**
Jugo: Insomnio, gargarismos, diurético	*Juice:* Insomnia, mouth gargle, diuretic
Cáscara: Transpiración, ayuda a hacer la digestión	*Peel:* Perspiration, aids in digestion
Cola de caballo (té)	**"Cola de caballo" (tea)**
Problemas de vías urinarias, depura la sangre	Urinary problems, "blood purification"
Tomillo (té)	**Thyme (tea)**
Tos ferina, dolor de estómago, pleurisia, bronquitis, amigdalitis, resfriados, abscesos, fiebre tifoidea	Whooping cough, stomach ache, pleurisy, bronchitis, tonsillitis, colds, abscess, typhoid fever
Diente de león (té)	**Dandelion (tea)**
Fiebre, ulceras, impuresas en la piel, acumulación de acido urico, gota, constipación, reumatismo	Fever, ulcers, skin impurities, uric acid buildup, gout, constipation, rheumatism
Granada	**Pomegranate (root and peel)**
Parasitosis intestinal	Intestinal parasitosis

Continued.

Table 4–1 Some Common Mexican and Hispanic Folk Remedies (Remedios Caseros)—cont'd

Spanish	English
Grosella	**Gooseberry**
Té: Laxante, descongestionante intestinal y del higado, reumatismo, gota	*Tea:* Laxative, liver and intestinal decongestant, skin infections, rheumatism, gout
Raíz: Acumulación de albumina	*Root:* Albumin buildup
Patatas asadas	**Baked potatoes (warm)**
Amigdalitas	Tonsillitis
Pelos de elote	**Corn silk**
Dolor al orinar	Painful urination
Nopal	**Prickly pear**
Diabetes	Diabetes
Lechuga (té)	**Lettuce (tea)**
Insomnio	Insomnia
Arnica	**Arnica**
Dolores musculares	Muscle pain
Borraja, sauco y eucaliptus	**Borage, elderberry, and eucalyptus (tea)**
Problemas respiratorios	Respiratory problems
Borraja y souco (té)	**Borage and elderberry (tea)**
Acelera la aparición de los sintomas de la varicela y acorta el curso de la enfermedad	Accelerates symptoms of chicken pox to shorten disease course
Hojas de guayabo	**Guava leaves (tea)**
Diarrea	Diarrhea

Table 4–1 Some Common Mexican and Hispanic Folk Remedies (Remedios Caseros)—cont'd

Spanish	English
Semillas de calabaza Parasitosis	**Pumpkin seed** Parasitosis
Romero (duchas vaginales) Tonicidad muscular	**Rosemary (vaginal douche)** Muscular tonicity
Magnolia Problemas cardiacos	**Magnolia (tea)** Heart problems
Alcanfor, alcohol, marihuana Artiritis	**Camphor, alcohol, marijuana** Arthritis
Chile verde Orzuelo	**Green chili (whole, cool, and moist)** Sty
Plátano maduro asado con mantequilla Laringo traqueo bronquitis	**Baked ripe banana with butter** Laryngotracheal bronchitis
Epazote Flatulencia	**Mexican tea** Flatulence
Azahar, valeriana Tranquilizante nervioso	**Citrus blossom, valerian (tea)** Nerve tranquilizer
Ricino Laxante, inductor del vomito	**Ricine (oil)** Laxative, induces vomiting
Digital Infermedades cardiacas	**Digitalis tea** Heart disease

not embrace a belief system, be it humanism, atheism, Buddhism, or any identified belief system, she/he may not be sensitive to the need that many patients have to be spiritually comforted during times of crisis. The percentage of individuals in the general population who claim a belief in a personal God is much greater than the percentage of health care providers, particularly physicians, who claim such a belief (Schreiber, 1991). It is clear that patients who do have an identified belief or value system experience less fear and have fewer complications when they are given access to individuals, rituals, or items that provide them with a sense of spiritual comfort and reassurance (McKee and Chappel, 1992). This occurs through a reduction of psychologic fear and, according to many patients' belief systems, through the comfort of a loving God. The majority of patients indicate that religious and spiritual beliefs are important to them, yet they do not feel that health care professionals are concerned with their spiritual needs (Anderson et al., 1993; Schreiber, 1991). Understanding the significance of patients' spiritual and religious beliefs can be helpful in understanding the meaning that a patient's illness or injury has to the patient, which may also affect the patient's recovery. For example, patients from a Southeast Asian background may believe that an illness is caused by angry spirits evoked by thoughts the patient has had or by an action he/she has taken. The health care provider who respects this philosophy may gain the trust of the patient. This trust facilitates the benefits for medical therapy when ritualistic religious practices to placate the spirits are performed according to the patient's community of belief (Gilman et al., 1992).

To assess whether patients need facilitation of spiritual well-being, the triage or health care professional should ask patients whether they have a belief system. While it is not realistic for health care professionals to be apprised of the significance of every body of religious belief, it is possible, when the patient states, "Yes, I am Muslim," to ask the patient whether his/her religious beliefs have ramifications for the patient's health care. If the patient responds in the affirmative, the professional should indicate that, whenever possible, the patient will be enabled to incorporate his/her beliefs into his/her health care. (However, triage nurses or health care providers must be sure that they can give this assurance, since at times the patient's religious beliefs may conflict with the treatment plan.)

Any concerns of families or patients that may involve medical, legal, or ethical dilemmas should be referred to the physician whose ultimate responsibility it is to discuss medical decisions. All providers should be willing to ask patients about their religious beliefs and whether they are in conflict with proposed care. Such conflict is most dramatically evident when blood transfusions are proposed for Jehovah's Witnesses, who may be at risk of separation from their church should they choose to receive a transfusion or to allow their child to undergo transfusion (Roy-Bornstein et al., 1994). In the past, transfusions were routinely ordered based on specific surgeries, whereas today there is a much more conservative approach to transfusion, since death precipitated by postsurgical anemia is quite rare (Kitchens, 1993). Triage nurses should not make the assumption that a patient will receive a blood transfusion based on his/her presentation or history, and all such questions should be deferred to the physician. However, it may be helpful to ascertain whether a patient has a signed card prohibiting the use of blood transfusions, since this has been legally upheld as a valid legal document that must be respected by health care providers (Rosam, 1991). It is the physician's role to write orders regarding transfusions, but it is the nurse's role to obtain information and provide documentation, if possible, and to be an advocate for the rights of the patient. If there is a lack of an advance directive or documentation indicating that the Jehovah's Witness patient wishes to deny transfusions, the presumption is that a transfusion should be administered only to render lifesaving treatment.

At times it may not be realistic for patients to practice religious rituals in a health care setting, but respect should be shown and provisions made when it is possible. If a patient indicates that he/she would like a Bible, it is not appropriate for a provider to state, ''This is a public hospital. We don't have Bibles here.'' It would be more helpful to state that Bibles are not readily available and that it would be best if the patient could have a family member or friend bring one to the hospital. Hospital chaplains are often ''on call'' for public hospitals and can be called to work with patients requesting spiritual comfort.

Hospital chaplains are educated in world religions and belief systems and can facilitate the patient's requests for specific spiritual comfort measures or help contact a religious mentor from the patient's religious community.

Although it is unrealistic for health care providers to be knowledgeable on all world religions or spiritual belief systems, it is enriching to professional practice to have a knowledge base that includes knowing which major religious beliefs can have an impact on patient care. For example, children of parents who do not believe in immunization or medical therapy may have infectious diseases such as pertussis that are not commonly seen in the general pediatric population (Etkind et al., 1992). If a triage nurse knows that a pediatric patient is associated with a religious group that does not allow immunization, he/she should interview the parents specifically regarding whether the child has received any immunizations, and the response to this query should be included in the triage record. Children of parents who do not believe in conventional Western medical care may have complications and may even die of chronic illness such as diabetes (Brahams, 1993). Patients who participate in religious practices that include changes in their normal health habits, such as fasting during Ramadan, as is done by many Muslims, may be

---

CASE REPORT 1

J.D. is a 48-year-old Kuwaiti-American man who was seen in the ED for acute abdominal pain. His workup indicated that he had an acute condition in the abdomen requiring emergency surgery. When the nurse asked the patient whether there was anything that would be helpful to him in relation to his Muslim beliefs, he requested time to face east toward Mecca and pray before she started his intravenous line. Although the nurse was pressed for time, she recognized the patient's right to practice his religion and receive the comfort it would provide him. The nurse requested that the patient use no more than 5 minutes if possible. When she returned, the patient thanked her and said, "Now I feel I can go to surgery at peace."

CASE REPORT 2

O.H., a 68-year-old Caucasian American woman, was diagnosed with adult-onset diabetes 1 month before arriving at triage with diabetic ketoacidosis. During the triage process the nurse discovered that the patient was noncompliant with her insulin regimen. The nurse asked the patient what she found difficult about taking her insulin, and she replied, "I'm a Seventh-Day Adventist and I find it so hard to take insulin, which comes from pork. I just can't make myself do it, even though it isn't against my beliefs; I've just never taken anything into my system that had anything to do with pork." The nurse recorded the patient's comments on the ED record and reassured the patient that alternatives compatible with her identified needs were available. The patient's insulin was switched to Humulin insulin beginning in the ED, and after discharge from the hospital the patient was compliant with her therapeutic regime.

CASE REPORT 3

A.M. was a 17-year-old Mexican girl who had paramedics to her home when she had a spontaneous abortion of a 5-month-old fetus. During the medics' treatment a Spanish-speaking medic asked the patient if she was Catholic. When she answered in the affirmative, the medic asked the patient if she would like the baby named and baptized. She nodded "yes" and said that the baby's name should be "Ignacio." The medic baptized "Ignacio," sprinkling water over him and saying, "I baptize you, Ignacio, in the name of the Father, Son, and Holy Ghost." Although not Catholic himself, the medic was aware of the belief of many Catholics that a baby who was not baptized would have a soul that would float through eternity and would not be united with its mother in heaven. The mother was greatly relieved and, although greatly upset by her loss, repeatedly thanked the medic for his kindness during the ambulance ride to the hospital.

affected by these practices, particularly when chronic health problems are present (Rashed, 1992). It is advisable to clarify with patients any special considerations related to their religion that the health care providers should be made aware of. This information should be recorded succinctly in the patient's record and highlighted when it has immediate impact on emergency care. The following case reports of patients with particular religious beliefs illustrate the importance of considering spiritual comfort during triage and emergency treatment of ill and injured patients.

Patients may not readily identify their spiritual needs, but when health care providers recognize that spirituality is an important component of their patient's overall health—whether it is identified as an individual belief of the patient about how the patient interacts with the universe or as a specific religious affiliation—they will be more likely to include the patient's spiritual well-being during the triage and interview process.

Specific considerations about various belief systems as they pertain specifically to triage and emergency care are listed in Table 4–2.

Situations that place the health care provider in a difficult position may arise. For example, she/he may be asked to participate in religious rituals or do things to comfort patients spiritually and psychologically, such as pray with them. The action taken by the professional should be determined by what that professional is comfortable with and by the policies of the agency for whom the individual works. Keeping the patient's best interests at heart and using support services and others significant to the patient to work with the individual help provide spiritual comfort without compromising the health care provider's time or ethics.

As professionals build their knowledge base of cultural issues in patient care, they will be better prepared to acknowledge and assess the ways in which patients' beliefs affect their health care. Sometimes health care providers may request that patients defer certain religious practices if they are disruptive to an environment in which other patients may be negatively affected. This is an uncommon situation and can often be avoided by incorporating the patient's spiritual needs into the plan of patient care.

Table 4–2 Religious Beliefs and Triage Practice

Belief system	Relevance to triage and emergency department
Atheism	Patients may request the presence of others significant to them during crisis to provide human comfort and a sense of peace.
Buddhism	Patients may believe that crisis is a result of wrong committed in present or past life. Many believe that if they are good, good will be done to them or a positive outcome will be their reward. Kindness from providers will be a comfort.
Catholicism	Some Catholics believe that the souls of infants who die and have not been baptized will float through eternity. Any layperson may baptize an infant with a sprinkle of water, saying ''I baptize you in the name of the Father, Son, and Holy Ghost.''
	Some Catholics who are critically ill may like to have a priest called to administer the Sacrament of the Sick and to talk with them.
	Some Catholics find that having rosary beads or prayer books is comforting.
Gypsies	Diseases are divided into non-Gypsy (*gaje*) diseases, which are treatable by Western practitioners, and Gypsy diseases, which must be treated by their own practitioners (*drabarni*). Disease may be thought to be caused by the evil eye.
	Some foods are thought to be lucky (pepper, salt, vinegar, garlic, and onions) and necessary for good health. Family presence is vital to reducing fear and the risk of agitation.*
Jehovah's Witness	Patients may request that members of their religious group be present to comfort and talk with them. If they have family

*From Southerland A: *West J Med* 157(3):276, 1992.

Continued.

Table 4–2 Religious Beliefs and Triage Practice—cont'd

Belief system	Relevance to triage and emergency department
	members who have at one time been Jehovah's Witnesses and have left the religion, the patients may have "shunned" them; patients may, during a time of crisis, wish to see a family member with whom they have chosen to no longer associate.
Judaism	There are varying degrees of religious orthodoxy and personal preference regarding religious practices. Some individuals with Jewish ethnicity do not practice Judaism, and patients should be asked whether they have religious beliefs that should be considered in the situation. Some might like to have the rabbi called. Some choose not to eat pork or shellfish.
Latter-day Saints (Mormon)	Bishops are considered spiritual leaders of the smallest unit of believers. They act to provide spiritual comfort during times of crisis, as well as advocating and arranging for the physical and social needs of the patient and family. The patient may wish to have the bishop or other friends or family who espouse Mormonism called during a time of crisis. Most do not use alcohol or consume caffeine.
Mien (non-Christian)	*Sip mmien* ceremonies conducted by a male head of household or a Mien specialist may be performed to appease angry ancestral spirits. Such ceremonies may involve the sacrifice of a domestic animal slaughtered by a packing-house in a manner consistent with ceremonial requirements. *Phat* is another ceremony whereby ancestral spirits are appeased in the treatment of ailments such as respiratory diseases or "soul fright." Cupping is also a common practice.

Table 4–2   Religious Beliefs and Triage Practice—cont'd

Belief system	Relevance to triage and emergency department
Muslim	Many Muslims maintain daily prayer habits that include praying thrice daily while facing east. Some also like to pray before interventions. Most choose not to eat pork. Certain religious holidays involve fasting.
Protestant	Many patients who indicate that they are ''Protestant'' may at one time have had a specific religious affiliation with a church group such as Methodism, and they may wish to have a minister from a particular Protestant church asked to visit them. Since there is a wide variety of Christian beliefs within Protestantism, it is best to ask patients in what way their identified religion is important to them and how it might relate to their crisis. Some patients might request a Bible or a hospital chaplain.
Seventh-day Adventist	A Protestant religion. The preceding recommendations given for Protestants also apply for this group. Many people espousing this religion do not consume alcohol, caffeine, or foods containing pork or shellfish or use tobacco in any form.
Southeast Asians (non-Christian)	Many believe that illness is a result of weak nerves or an imbalance of yin and yang, an obstruction of *chi* (life energy), disharmony with nature, a curse, or a punishment for immorality. Coining, cupping, and moxibustion may be practiced. Herbal remedies are commonly used.

REFERENCES

Anderson JM, Anderson LJ, Felsenthal G: Pastoral needs and support within an inpatient rehabilitation unit, *Arch Phys Med Rehabil* 74(6):574, 1993.

Asnis DS, Saltzman HP, Melchert A: Shark oil pneumonia: an overlooked entity, *Chest* 103(3):976, 1993.

Berry RG, Collymore VA: Otitis externa and facial cellulitis from Oriental ear cleaners, *West J Med* 158(5):536, 1993.

Brahams D: Religious objection versus parental duty, *Lancet* 342(88881):1189, 1993.

Brod M, Heurtin-Roberts S: Older Russian emigrés and medical care, *West J Med* 157(3):333, 1992.

Buchwald D, Panwala S, Hooton TM: Use of traditional health practices by Southeast Asian refugees in a primary care clinic, *West J Med* 156(5):507, 1992.

Capobianco DJ, Brazis PW, Fox TP: Proximal-muscle weakness induced by herbs, *N Engl J Med* 329(19):1430, 1993 (letter).

Cohn MJ, Cohen AJ: RADCOM: a computerized translation device for use during fluoroscopic examination of non-English-speaking patients, *Am J Roentgenol* 162(2):455, 1994.

D'Avanzo CE: Barriers to health care for Vietnamese refugees, *J Prof Nurs* 8(4):245, 1992.

Diaz-Gilbert M: Caring for culturally diverse patients, *Nursing* 23(10):44, 1993.

Etkind P, Lett SM, Macdonald PD et al: Pertussis outbreaks in groups claiming religious exemptions to vaccinations, *Am J Dis Child* 146(2):173, 1992.

Garty BZ: Garlic burns, *Pediatrics* 91(3):658, 1993.

Giger JN, Davidhizar RE: *Transcultural nursing,* St Louis, 1995, Mosby.

Giger JN, Davidhizar RE, Turner G: Black American folk medicine health care beliefs: implication for nursing plans of care, *ABNF* 3(2):42, 1992.

Gilman SC, Justice J, Saepharn K et al: Use of traditional and modern health services by Laotian refugees, *West J Med* 157(3):310, 1992.

Grossman D: Enhancing your "cultural competence," *Am J Nurs* 94(7):58, 1994.

Haffner L: Translation is not enough: interpreting in a medical setting, *West J Med* 157(3):255, 1992.

Hufnagel TJ, Schein OD: Suppurative keratitis from herbal ocular preparation, *Am J Ophthalmol* 113(6):722, 1992.

Isaacman DJ, Purvis K, Gyuro J, et al: Standardized instructions: do they improve communication of discharge information from the emergency department? *Pediatrics* 89(6, Pt 2):1204, 1992.

Jolly BT, Scott JL, Feied CF et al: Functional illiteracy among emergency department patients: a preliminary study, *Ann Emerg Med* 22(3):573, 1993.

Kassler WJ, Blanc P, Greenblatt R: The use of medicinal herbs by human immunodeficiency virus–infected patients. *Arch Intern Med* 151(11):2281, 1991.

Kew J, Morris C, Aihie A et al: Arsenic and mercury intoxication due to Indian ethnic remedies, *Br Med J* 306(6876), 1993.

Kitchens CS: Are transfusions overrated? Surgical outcome of Jehovah's Witnesses, *Am J Med* 94(2):117, 1993.

Markowitz SB, Nunez CM, Klitzman S et al: Lead poisoning due to hai ge fen: the porphyrin content of individual erythrocytes, *JAMA* 271(12):932, 1994.

McKee DD, Chappel JN: Spirituality and medical practice, *J Fam Pract* 35(2):201, 205, 1992.

Morgan PP: Illiteracy can have major impact on patients' understanding of health care information, *Can Med Assoc J* 148(7):1196, 1993.

Nussinovitch M, Amir J, Varsano I: Chemical pneumonia and dermatitis caused by kerosene, *Clin Pediatr* 31(9):574, 1992.

Ponder A, Lehman LB: 'Coining' and 'coning': an unusual complication of unconventional medicine, *Neurology* 44(4):774, 1994.

Rashed AH: The fast of Ramadan, *Br Med J* 306(6826)521, 1992.

Rosam ED: Patients' rights and the role of the emergency physician in the management of Jehovah's Witnesses, *Ann Emerg Med* 20(10):1150, 1991.

Roy-Bornstein C, Sagor LD, Roberts KB: Treatment of a Jehovah's Witness with immune globulin: case of a child with Kawasaki syndrome, *Pediatrics* 94(1):112, 1994.

Schreiber K: Religion in the physician-patient relationship, *JAMA* 266(21):3062, 3066, 1991.

Sutherland A: Gypsies and health care, *West J Med* 157(3):276, 1992.

Uba L: Cultural barriers to health care for Southeast Asian refugees, *Public Health Rep* 107(5):544, 1992.

RECOMMENDED READING

Geissler E: *Pocket guide to cultural assessment,* St Louis, 1994, Mosby.

Giger JN, Davidhizar RE: *Transcultural nursing,* St Louis, 1995, Mosby.

Perharic L, Shaw D, Murray V: Toxic effects of herbal medicines and food supplements, *Lancet* 342(8864):180, 1993.

5 | The Patient Interview and General Appearance

Patient triaging is most often performed in an emergency department (ED) where patients are coming to the triage nurse with a variety of complaints. It is difficult, particularly when there is a high volume of patients, to rapidly switch attention from one patient to the next when their needs and complaints vary widely. Moving from the assessment of a woman with a threatened abortion to a young man complaining of hearing voices requires composure and a systematic plan to obtain answers to questions that are appropriate and necessary for a concise yet complete triage history.

Medical problems and traumatic injuries must always be approached using a systematic plan for the triage interview and physical assessment. The chief complaint and general appearance of the patient arriving for triage provide initial guidance for the focus of the triage assessment and may be sufficient in some instances for determining the patient's acuity level.

CHIEF COMPLAINT

The chief complaint is the patient's reason for seeking emergency care. The triage interviewer records the chief complaint in the patient's own words. It is necessary to be systematic and efficient at interviewing patients about their chief complaints. A number of methods are used for systematically obtaining information about a patient's chief complaint. It is best to use the same acronym or method consistently, to avoid omitting critical questions.

When patients arrive at triage, they are normally asked why they are seeking care. The patient's *first* response should be recorded and considered when determining whether the patient needs to be immediately triaged or can wait. It may be necessary to ask key questions after hearing the patient's chief complaint. For example, if a patient says she/he needs to be seen because she/he hurt a leg playing basketball, the triage professional must determine how badly the patient was hurt when the incident occurred, and whether ice and elevation of the injured extremity are immediately advised. Individuals who appear to have a simple sprain can receive first aid and wait their turn to be seen, whereas individuals with excruciating pain and an open fracture must be fully triaged immediately. Critical questions that must be asked in triage to assist in determining the patient's acuity level are listed in Box 5–1.

The time and manner of onset of the patient's chief complaint are determined by asking, ''When did this occur?'' or ''When did you notice the pain first started?'' If the patient indicates that the problem has been chronic over a period of weeks or months, the interviewer makes note of this and also records the patient's statement regarding when the problem was severe or bothersome enough that she/he felt she/he should seek emergency care.

BOX 5–1	Key Triage Questions Regarding a Patient's Chief Complaint

- When did the problem occur?
- How did the problem manifest?
- Do you have any ideas about what may have caused this problem?
- Can you describe how you feel?
- If there is pain, can you tell me if the pain radiates anywhere?
- How severe is the problem? (Ask about how the problem has affected the individual's capacity to perform activities of daily living, work, or sleep. If the problem is pain, ask the individual how severe the pain is on a scale of 1 to 10, with 10 being ''the worst pain ever felt or imagined.''
- Is this problem continuous, or does it come and go?
- Have you noticed a pattern associated with this problem?
- Can you describe any other symptoms you feel are associated with this problem?
- Is there anything you have done, taken, or used that has improved this problem? Has any remedy been effective in helping you feel better or feel that your problem is improved?

The manner of onset of the patient's problem should be elicited in an open-ended question format (i.e., "Tell me how you first noticed this problem.") The interviewer is interested in whether the problem had a sudden or gradual onset; this may be determined by asking the patient specifically whether the problem came on suddenly or gradually, but asking open-ended questions allows the patient to reveal key information that often provides clues to the causes of the problem. It may become apparent quite early in the interview process that the patient arrives with a reason for being seen that is not the true "chief complaint" or most pressing concern. For example, sometimes a patient arrives with a vague request. The patient may state, "I need an all-over check" when her/his true concern may be worries about having contracted a sexually transmissible disease (STD). The interviewer must record the patient's words within quotation marks and use intuition in deciding whether it is best to ask the patient if she/he is also seeking care for a more specific concern or to allow the ED or primary health care provider to discuss the patient's specific concerns.

In addition to using intuition, the triage interviewer makes the decision about how quickly to press the patient about the "real" chief complaint based on the facility's policy for seeing patients with nonurgent problems that might need to be triaged elsewhere such as to a clinic for treatment of an STD. Sometimes the triage professional uses personal judgment based on what she/he feels is best for the patient as a human being. For example, if a 17-year-old man requests "an all-over check" and confides that he is really concerned about having contracted an STD, the triage nurse may know that the ED "triages out" patients with the chief complaint of STD for care at an STD clinic. However, if the interviewer discovers that the patient will not go to an STD clinic if triaged out (because of fear or transportation problems, for example), the triage nurse sometimes manipulates the triage record to indicate that the patient has an "urgent" need to be seen, rather than a "nonurgent" need based on symptoms such as "severe discomfort." Although this practice is not condoned, this dilemma is prevalent, and the ethical aspects of patient care as they affect triage policies and practice in EDs must be considered.

Once the triage interviewer has determined the patient's

chief complaint and its time and manner of onset, the interviewer is ready to move on to other key questions that will elucidate the patient's problem. The *PQRST* mnemonic provides a format for questioning patients about their complaints. It is a systematic approach, as follows, that enables the triage nurse to be consistent in interviewing all patients.

Precipitating factors. Patients should be asked about what they feel may have caused the problem. The response gives valuable information not only about feasible precipitating factors but also about the patient's perceptions. If the patient is unable to provide information about what may have caused the problem, specific, closed-ended questions should be asked that are pertinent to the chief complaint. For example, if a patient arrives with a chief complaint such as ''I'm experiencing an allergic reaction,'' the interviewer, having determined the time and manner of the reaction, asks whether the patient knows what precipitated the allergic reaction (i.e., ''Do you have any idea what caused this allergic reaction?''). If the patient is unaware of what evoked the allergic response, the examiner asks specific questions to determine whether the patient was exposed to an insect, nuts, new soaps, fabrics, or other relevant potential allergens. Knowing what questions are relevant to the chief complaint requires a broad knowledge base and understanding of which precipitating factors are likely according to the chief complaint, general appearance, and problem-specific triage examination.

Palliative factors. Patients should be questioned about whether they have done anything or taken any medication, folk medicines, or home remedies to improve their condition. The triage nurse also asks whether the act or remedy was effective in reducing or relieving, even temporarily, the patient's symptoms.

Quality. Patients are asked about the nature of their chief complaint. This most often relates to the nature of pain. For example, patients are asked if they can describe their pain. If they are unable to do so because they do not understand how to answer the question, the interviewer then asks about the quality of the pain in a closed-ended manner (Fig. 5–1).

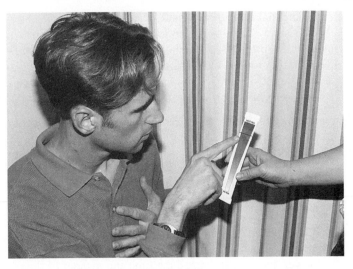

Fig. 5–1 Visual tools to assist patients in quantifying the severity of their pain are helpful for triage adjuncts.

For example, the patient is asked, ''Is the pain stabbing, squeezing, crushing, or aching or can you describe or think of any other word that can describe what you are feeling?'' Once a patient has adjectives to choose from, it is often easier to state the nature of the pain or discomfort. Discerning the quality of pain is often useful in determining whether the patient's problem is visceral or superficial and can give clues about the patient's acuity and the possible origin of the problem. A patient who has a complaint other than pain should be asked to describe the nature of the problem, and the response should be recorded.

Radiation and location. The patient is asked to indicate the specific location of the problem or symptoms. This is helpful in judging, in some instances, whether the problem is nonurgent, urgent, or emergent. For example, a patient who complains of chest pain and who can point to the location of chest pain with one finger, stating that it is sharp and bothersome, is most likely not experiencing an emergent cardiac problem. On the other hand, a patient who describes crushing chest pain and who indicates the location of pain with a fist to the sternum (positive Levine's sign) is most likely experiencing a critical cardiac event that must be triaged as "emergent." In addition to asking the patient to specifically indicate the location of the pain or symptoms, the interviewer should ask whether the pain travels or radiates and if so, ask the patient to indicate where. If the patient seems unclear about how to respond, the interviewer specifically asks the patient whether the pain or problem is also experienced in other areas, specifically indicating the area. For example, if patient is having abdominal pain, the patient should be asked whether the pain radiates across the abdomen or the epigastrium, to the flank area, down the legs, to the chest, or in one or both shoulders. According to the knowledge base of the interviewer, the index of suspicion for a number of causes of the patient's symptoms will rise; the patient's acuity status is determined most safely when the information from the triage interview is considered in conjunction with key factors such as vital signs.

Severity. The patient is questioned about the severity of symptoms. If the patient is in pain, she/he is asked to describe the severity of the pain on a scale of 1 to 10, with 10 being the most pain the patient has ever experienced or imagined. If the severity of the pain varies because it is intermittent, the patient is asked how severe the pain is at its worst (how highly it rates) and how severe it is (how highly it is rated) at the time of the interview. If the patient has difficulty comprehending how to rate the pain on a scale of 1 to 10, the patient can be asked to state whether it is less than or greater than "5," or moderate pain. A scale using faces to illustrate degrees of pain is useful for patients whose first language is not English or for those who cannot describe the severity of the pain easily in words, such as children. It is important, if a pain scale of faces is used, that patients understand what is being asked of them. If the patient does not have pain but has other symptoms, she/he can be asked to describe the effect of the symptoms and problems on activities of daily living. Specific questions related to determining severity should also be included. For example, if a woman complains of vaginal bleeding, the examiner asks about the number of pads or tampons, or both, the patient is using per hour. This information, in addition to other triage information gathered during the triage assessment, helps the interviewer determine the appropriate triage acuity level of the patient.

Time. The patient is asked about time factors relevant to the chief complaint, including whether the symptom(s) has (have) been continuous or intermittent and if there is a pattern related to the symptoms. This should be done in a brief manner with the understanding that a more detailed interview will be performed by the health care providers who will treat the patient.

The PQRST format for interviewing a patient about the chief complaint is intended as a framework and should be guided by the interviewer's professional background and knowledge and the patient's general appearance and apparent acuity. If a patient comes to triage with an obviously critical problem, the triage professional may choose to immediately access care for the patient and allow the health care providers to obtain information that is normally obtained during the triage interview. This is the best action the triage nurse can take for a patient with an emergent problem, since the patient's primary need is for immediate, appropriate care. It is always better to err on the side of caution and triage a patient who is severely ill or injured directly into the ED than to delay care in triage.

GENERAL APPEARANCE

In addition to the discernment of triage acuity based on the patient's chief complaint, rapid triage decisions are also made based on the patient's general appearance. Most often, a triage acuity designation is determined by the patient's triage history, general appearance, and vital signs and a brief physical assessment. Before obtaining general information and clinical measurements, the nurse may decide to take action based on the patient's general appearance (Fig. 5–2). The complete components and the merit of evaluating a patient's general appearance are well defined and discussed in textbooks on physical assessment. Typically, a health professional considers one or more of

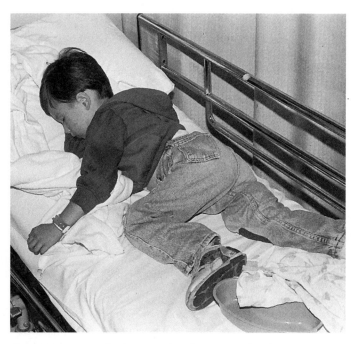

Fig. 5–2 Diminished activity level is a critical indication in general appearance of children.

the characteristics of the patient's general appearance that are listed in Box 5–2.

Impressions formed on the basis of evaluating an individual's general appearance are useful for determining acuity and recording a partial impression of the patient's mental status. The general appearance of an individual is determined by many factors, such as health status, acuity of the illness or injury for which the patient is seeking medical attention in triage, personality, culture, economic factors, and emotional status. In the triage system the triage professional understands these factors and uses those parts of the general appearance that are most useful in determining the patient's triage category and immediate needs. Only the most relevant characteristics of a patient's general appearance are usually included in the triage record.

| BOX 5–2 | **Characteristics of General Appearance** |

- Level of consciousness
- Obvious signs of distress or disease
- Gait ability and comfort: use of aids if present
- Appropriateness of weight for height and developmental status
- Facial expressions and mannerisms
- General hygiene
- Appropriateness of clothing for weather, whether clothing is clean and well fitting
- Striking features and deformities (Fig. 5–3)
- Language and speech: logic and articulation

Obvious Signs of Distress

A patient may exhibit obvious signs of distress as a result of a physical problem. Depending on the origin of the symptoms and the level of threat concurrently associated with the patient's distress, this problem may be sufficient for emergent triage. The triage nurse should consider general signs of airway compromise or respiratory distress as requiring emergent triage. The general appearance of an individual with airway emergencies may include cyanosis, pallor or ashen skin, tachypnea or bradypnea, dyspnea, stridor or crowing noise, agitation or anxiety, obvious use of accessory muscles, and nasal flaring. This appearance may be an indication that the patient is worn out and is no longer compensating for a critical oxygenation problem. If an individual is able to speak, the nurse should note the ability to speak in sentences.

Individuals who seek medical attention in triage with obvious signs of circulation difficulties may exhibit many of the signs of airway and breathing emergencies. In addition, the patient may appear confused, have a diminished level of alertness, or appear pale and diaphoretic. Some individuals point to or clutch the chest, which may be an obvious sign of circulatory distress. Circulation crises may also occur in the form of excessive bleeding. The wounds of patients with obvious bleeding

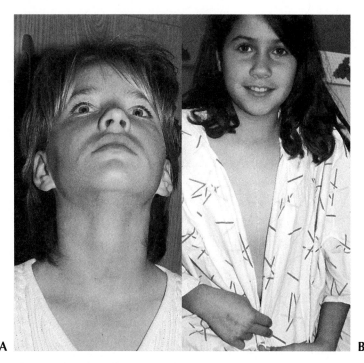

A   B

Fig. 5–3   Striking features such as surgical scars may be directly relevant to the patient's chief complaint. **A,** Tracheostomy scar. **B,** Sternotomy scar.

must be immediately evaluated, but these patients should not be triaged as emergent on the basis of obvious bleeding, since wounds that occur in highly vascular areas such as scalp may bleed profusely but can be controlled with pressure; they do not always result in hypovolemia. A full evaluation is appropriate for the best triage decision. Patients with pulsatile blood flow resulting from arterial injuries, however, may arrive at triage with this obvious vascular emergency and are triaged as emergent; a full triage assessment is appropriately deferred.

Patients with pain in the head and neck find it difficult to use common coping mechanisms such as distraction for dealing with pain because the pain prevents the individual from being able to think clearly enough to focus on anything besides the pain. Although complaints of the head and neck and those involving neurologic symptoms often do not have life-threatening implications, because they are so distressing to the patient the patient is likely to have a highly emotional affect and demand immediate attention.

Great patience and empathy are required of the triage nurse when triaging many patients with migraine headaches, toothaches, and neck and back pain, yet it is comforting to the patient when a triage nurse indicates that he/she feels it is unfortunate that the patient has severe discomfort.

Gait: Comfort and Ability

The patient's ability to ambulate and the limitations he/she may have during ambulation are observed. Specific gait evaluation is the responsibility of the health care provider, but the triage professional records whether the patient ambulates easily or notes the presence of an antalgic limp. Limitations to easy ambulation other than musculoskeletal injuries should also be recorded, such as severe body pain (e.g., pain in the abdomen), extreme fatigue, dizziness, nausea, or other symptoms. In the absence of injuries the inability to ambulate is especially critical in children, whose decrease in activity may indicate a serious health crisis. As the triage professional interviews the patient to determine for severity of symptoms, onset of ambulation difficulties should also be appraised and a problem-specific examination performed.

Appropriateness of Weight for Height and Developmental Status

Making a general observation about the patient's weight in proportion to height is particularly useful in determining the pediatric patient's acuity status and potential problems such as dehydration or failure to thrive. Although it is not the role of the triage professional to make medical diagnoses, it can be helpful to note the patient's general appearance when the patient is excessively underweight or overweight, especially in conjunction with signs of dehydration or fluid retention. A patient who appears emaciated must be carefully questioned about preexisting or acute medical problems in conjunction with or in addition to the chief complaint. The patient is asked whether there have been recent changes in weight, since this is as crucial as disproportionate height and weight. The patient with recent weight changes is also asked for her/his impressions about why the change has occurred, since not all weight change is related to illness but may result from a weight loss diet plan.

Facial Expressions and Mannerisms

Observation of the patient's facial expression may be useful in validating an examiner's impression about the patient's level of distress (Fig. 5–4). However, it is also important to remember that many patients in acute distress do not reveal their discomfort or distress by their facial expressions. Cultural and individual variants must be considered. The patient's facial expression may also be useful in detecting risk of violent behavior, agitation, or mental health or emotional crisis. Assessing and recording incongruence among facial expressions, manner-

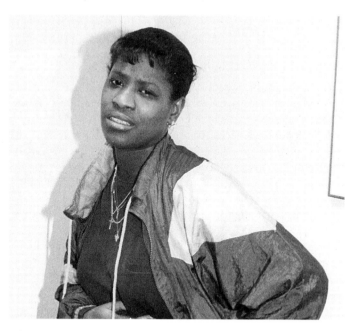

Fig. 5–4 Facial expressions are useful indicators in triage.

isms, and the patient's chief complaint is important. This is true for family members or significant others as well as for patients. For example, a flat or detached affect between an abusive care provider and a patient is often paramount in detecting abuse.

Mannerisms exhibited by patients during observation of their general appearance, such as obvious tics, spasms, compulsive behaviors, or other mannerisms, should be recorded.

General Hygiene

Observations about the patient's general hygiene are relevant to neurologic status, mental status, and safety. Normally, general hygiene is not mentioned unless there are obvious deficits in this area. It is most helpful, when there are problems with hygiene, to specifically describe the deficits so that a general statement of poor hygiene does not reflect the interviewer's values but is clearly validated by objective observations. This is especially important in issues of conservatorship or abuse. Notes may include visual and olfactory descriptors of the hygienic condition of the hair, nails, clothing, teeth, or skin. Qualifying statements made by care providers or the patient themselves regarding poor hygiene should also be included in the record.

Appropriateness of Clothing

Observations of the appropriateness of the patient's clothing for the weather and how well the clothing fits can be relevant to the patient's neurologic, mental, and economic status. When a patient does not have access to necessary clothing because of economic difficulties, the triage nurse, if time permits, may provide information about community agencies that can provide clothing the patient needs. Clothing that is ill fitting or inappropriate for the weather may indicate neglect in the pediatric or geriatric patient. The triage nurse specifically records what the patient is wearing and qualifying statements made by the care provider or patient regarding the patient's dress. Community resources discussed in triage should be recorded on the discharge record so that the patient has a written reference for agencies where they may seek assistance.

Striking Features and Obvious Deformities

Any notable feature or characteristic about a patient that is striking may be noteworthy in the triage record. Such features may include obvious deformities such as avulsed lacerations, ecchymoses, or hematomas. Asymmetries such as those seen in Bell's palsy or chronic hemiparesis may also be relevant. Information significant to the patient's history that is newly obtained when asking the patient about a striking feature should be added to the appropriate section in the triage record (e.g., "past medical problems or conditions").

LANGUAGE AND SPEECH: LOGIC AND ARTICULATION

Speech is the articulation of sounds. Language is the expression of thoughts and ideas. Patients with deficits or abnormalities in speech or language, or both, may have problems with hearing, cranial nerves, or receptive or expressive language centers in the brain. Furthermore, acute neurologic or neuromuscular problems or the effects of medications, street drugs, or alcohol may be evident in speech and language. Notations about the general pattern of speech and language are usually reserved for patients with deficits or abnormalities in this area. It is important to record speech and language problems concisely because they validate the professional's general summary of the patient's distress or discomfort level. For example, a patient with a cardiovascular accident may be observed to attempt speech but have the ability to produce only repetitive sounds. Both the patient's effort and result should be noted in the triage record. If speech is slurred and other observations indicate cerebellar problems, such as an ataxic gait, these observations should also be noted in the record.

LEVEL OF AWARENESS

When neurologic disorders or symptoms are probable, it is helpful to indicate the patient's level of awareness both in short, descriptive terms and through use of objective tools such as the Glasgow Coma Scale. The triage professional establishes the patient's presentation in triage. Any changes indicating either improvement or deterioration are measured against the triage evaluation. Descriptors that may be used include the following: alert, stuporous, lethargic, semicomatose, and comatose. Efforts to arouse the nonalert patient should be recorded. In the patient who is verbally responsive, orientation to time, place, and person should also be established and assessed.

SUMMARY

A swift, thorough interview of a patient who arrives at triage in an emergency situation is performed most efficiently when the triage professional has a concise format for the triage interview. Professionals are aware that the patient's chief complaint may not be the true, pressing health concern for which she/he is seeking health care; nonetheless, information on the presenting complaint is essential. Ethical dilemmas that affect the assignment of the most appropriate acuity level must be revealed and discussed.

Assessing the patient's general appearance helps the triage professional determine the most appropriate acuity level for an individual. It can also be helpful to record key points about a patient's general appearance when issues of neglect or abuse are immediately evident. Recording findings about general appearance validates information in an subjective summary by providing objectively observed data and details. Only abnormal, dramatic, or striking characteristics of general appearance, such as signs of obvious distress, disease, or deformities, are recorded.

RECOMMENDED READING

Rowe JA: Triage assessment tool, *J Emerg Nurs* 18(6):540, 1992.
Wagner B et al: Triage assessment and nursing record, *J Emerg Nurs* 19(4):340, 1993.

6 | Neurologic and Head and Neck Problems

The brain is the most important organ of the body. It is the command center for all body system functions and enables perception, thinking, and movement—activities that all give protection, meaning, and pleasure to human life.

Neurologic symptoms and head injuries can be uncomfortable for the patient and frightening for both patient and significant others. Head injuries take priority for immediate evaluation. Concern for the patient's fears and discomfort should be immediately communicated, to help relax the patient at the onset of the triage process and enable a thorough triage assessment. Care must be taken to listen for critical cues indicating emergent problems, and the neurologic assessment done in triage should err if necessary on the side of detail rather then brevity.

NEUROLOGIC PROBLEMS
Headaches

Patients who complain of headache may have this symptom as a chief complaint, or it may be mentioned as an accompanying symptom to another, more pressing concern (chief complaint). Patients with a chief complaint of ''headache'' should not automatically be triaged as ''nonurgent'' or ''urgent'' based on the assumption that headache is not a significant or life-threatening problem. The majority of headaches are benign; however, careful assessment is crucial for detecting cues that are present when a critical neurologic emergency is concurrent with headache.

Headaches may be primary (have no underlying cause), and these are the most common; or secondary (have their origin in structural or physiologic disease, e.g., cardiovascular accident, meningeal irritation, or intracranial pressure changes and facial, cervical, systemic, or traumatic causes) (Weiss, 1993).

Patients with a headache should be allowed to describe

BOX 6–1	**Key Questions To Ask Patients With Headache**

- When did it start? Did it come on suddenly or gradually?
- What do you think may have brought it on?
- Can you describe how it feels?
- Is it continuous or does it come and go?
- Show me where it feels the worst and everywhere you feel it.
- On a scale of 1 to 10, with 10 being the worst headache you've ever felt, how bad is it right now?
- Have you taken any medication, including any over-the-counter medications such as aspirin or acetaminophen, to try to make the headache go away?
- Have you tried using anything such as ice or any home remedies?
- Do you have a history of migraines or headaches? If so, who has treated you for these in the past and what treatment has been used? Have you experienced relief from any treatment in the past?
- How often do you get headaches?

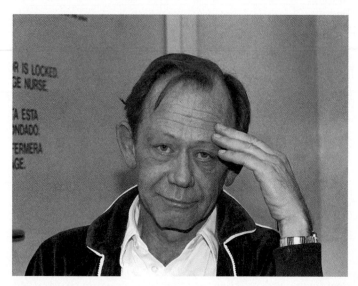

Fig. 6–1   Ask the patient to indicate the location and radiation of pain.

their problem before closed-ended questions are asked (Box 6–1). Time of onset of the headache should be recorded, as should manner of onset (e.g., sudden or gradual), quality of pain (squeezing, pulsating, pressure, stabbing, and the like), location and radiation (Fig. 6–1) (record according to the bones of the skull and muscles of the head and neck), severity (on a scale of 1 to 10, with 10 being the most pain ever experienced, also known as a "1 to 10 severity scale"), duration since onset (continuous or intermittent), and relieving factors (including home remedies or medications). It is important to know whether the patient has a history of headaches and, if so, who has treated the headaches in the past and what has been successful in alleviating the symptom. Another important area to explore with the patient is what may have precipitated the headache (Box 6–2). This question should be asked in an open-ended fashion, but possible precipitants may be mentioned and asked about if there is a suspicion that an identifiable factor may be present. Identifying the cause is helpful so that emergency department (ED) personnel can treat the headache and, if possible, the cause as well. Treatment may include appropriate referral to agencies that can help provide basic needs when the patient has inadequate resources. Identifying headache precipitants can also be useful in patient teaching, particularly when the patients may have prior knowledge, for example, regarding the links between inadequate food or fluid intake and headache. This particular cause of headache is often seen in adolescents.

BOX 6–2	**Precipitants to Headache**

- Inadequate sleep
- Inadequate food or fluid intake
- Use of or withdrawal from alcohol or drugs
- Noxious chemical exposure, e.g., fumes
- Stress
- Trauma to the head or history of such trauma
- Hypertension

BOX 6–3	**Symptoms of Increased Intracranial Pressure**

- Headache
- Nausea and vomiting
- Lethargy
- Diplopia
- Transient visual difficulty

Associated symptoms and problems the patient with a headache should be questioned about include sinus problems, fever, vision problems (last eye examination), photophobia, nausea, and vomiting. Headache may herald increased intracranial pressure (ICP), a potentially life-threatening neurologic emergency, and the triage nurse should be familiar with the cardinal symptoms of increased ICP (Box 6–3). Patients suspected of having problems with elevated ICP should be triaged as "emergent."

Presentations that should result in emergent or immediate triage designation include a report of a sudden-onset, extremely severe headache, often expressed as "the worst headache I've ever had in my life." The concern with this type of headache is that there may be a subdural hematoma, hemorrhage (subarachnoid or other), or acute hydrocephalus. A patient's use of the phrase "the worst headache I've ever had in my life" in describing a headache is sufficient for considering the condition emergent or immediate in the need to be diagnosed. The pattern of symptoms may be as important as one initial complaint or key phrase that is recognized during the history-taking process of triage.

Subdural hematomas are often fatal because they may go unrecognized while the ICP is increasing as the hematoma expands, a process that may occur immediately after onset of the hematoma or in a period of more than 2 weeks. The chronic variety occurs most frequently in infants, elderly persons, and alcoholic or demented individuals. Cues in the history that the triage nurse may detect in patients with this problem include

| BOX 6–4 | Symptoms of Subdural Hematoma |

- Persistent headache
- Drowsiness
- Progressive personality changes

persistent headache, drowsiness, and progressive personality changes (Box 6–4) (Donner, 1993).

Of great concern is the headache that is accompanied by fever and neck stiffness. This type of headache may be indicative of meningitis. Meningitis is often viral and not life threatening, although patients with viral meningitis may have major complications leading to learning, motor, or sensory disabilities and possibly death (Coderre, 1989). It is important to watch for signs of increased ICP (see Box 6–3). Although treatment for viral meningitis is mainly supportive and symptom based, accurate assessment is the key to patient recovery. Bacterial meningitis is often lethal; it is contagious, and it should be treated aggressively and immediately. Patients with acute meningococcemia may die within an hour of onset. The hallmarks of this infection include the classic symptoms of meningitis and a vascular rash of petechiae or purpura. Rapid assessment and early intervention are crucial to the survival of patients with meningococcemia (Box 6–5). Presenting signs and symptoms resemble those of common upper respiratory infections, beginning with fever, malaise, headache, muscle or joint pain, and gastrointestinal symptoms. There is also a history of irritability and decreased feeding in pediatric patients for up to 24 hours before presentation for medical care. Physical signs of a critical progression of the disease include a temperature of more than 40° Celsius, characteristic skin lesions, profound hypotension, tachycardia, poor peripheral perfusion, respiratory distress, cyanosis, and rapidly diminishing level of consciousness followed by coma and, too often, death (Jenkins, 1992).

Meningitis in the older adult is increasing, although the overall incidence of the disease in the United States is decreasing. The usual signs are neither as specific nor as sensitive

| BOX 6–5 | **Signs and Symptoms of Bacterial Meningitis** |

Early

- Headache, fever, malaise, muscle and joint pain
- Irritability, gastrointestinal upset
- Decreased appetite

Late

- Fever (temperature of more than 40° C)
- Macular, petechial, or purpuric skin rash
- Profound hypotension, poor peripheral perfusion
- Respiratory distress, cyanosis
- Diminished level of consciousness

as they are in younger patients, and since mortality and morbidity rates are high in elderly patients with this disease, the triage nurse must be particularly astute in watching for cues to this disease in older patients (Choi, 1992).

When dealing with patients suspected of having meningococcemia, care providers need to remember that it is contagious through respiratory droplets: a mask should be worn by all those coming into direct contact with the patient.

The triage physical assessment of the patient with headache or any neurologic complaint begins with vital signs. Presence of fever may increase the triage nurse's index of suspicion for meningitis or other infectious processes. Attention to blood pressure is necessary, since significant or chronic hypertension, such as hypertensive crisis, may be a precipitant to headache. Conversely, an elevated blood pressure may be a result of headache pain. Blood pressure in all patients should be reevaluated prior to discharge, and a reminder to perform this reassessment in the ED may be given by the triage nurse. In patients with headache who have increased ICP the triage nurse may detect a triad of vital sign changes known as Cushing's reflex: bradycardia, elevated blood pressure, and a widened pulse pressure, specifically, an increase in systolic pressure with lowering or

BOX 6–6	**Cushing's Reflex in Patients With Increased Intracranial Pressure**

- Bradycardias (heart rate ranging from 50 to 60 beats per minute)
- Elevated blood pressure: Elevated systolic pressure with a slight elevation or lowering of the diastolic pressure
- Slowed respiratory rate

slight elevation of diastolic pressure and a slowing of the respiratory rate (Box 6–6). Although Cushing's reflex is not always seen in the presence of increased ICP, an astute realization that the patient has the defined characteristics of this phenomenon is helpful and should result in emergent triage designation.

Assessment of pupil size, equality, and reaction to light is important; special attention should be given to equality of pupil size. Although anisocoria is a normal finding in a small percentage of patients, it should be considered highly significant unless it is verified as chronic and normal for the patient, since this abnormality may signify an acute neurologic emergency.

Range of motion of the head and neck should be assessed when meningitis is suspected, with particular attention to limitation and pain during flexion of the neck. If the patient has drainage from the nose or ears, the fluid may be tested for glucose level to screen for the presence of cerebrospinal fluid (CSF). The triage nurse often has no time to perform this last procedure, however, and recording the presence and characteristics of such fluid is sufficient. Recommended physical assessment measures to be performed on patients with a chief complaint of headache are listed in Box 6–7.

The triage nurse must have a solid understanding of the signs and symptoms of a variety of neurologic problems associated with headaches, not to diagnose the patient, but to detect gross abnormalities that enable an appropriate triage designation. Common, critical headache presentations are summarized in Box 6–8.

Even with astute concern for the subtle nuances of headache and other neurologic symptoms it is possible for serious

BOX 6–7	Physical Assessment of Patients with Headache

- Evaluation for fever
- Attention to blood pressure and pulse pressure
- Attention to pulse rate for variations from normal
- Checking of pupil size, equality, and response to light
- Recording of the presence and characteristics of any fluid draining from the nose or ears

BOX 6–8	Headache Causes and Patterns of Presentation

- Tension: Diffuse, steady, occipital or frontal, and "bandlike"
- Migraines: Periodic, throbbing, severe, frequently unilateral, and often over the eye(s); photophobia and sensitivity to sound are common, as are nausea and vomiting.
- Cluster headaches: Very painful, knifelike, unilateral, and over the eye
- Brain tumor: Of patients with brain tumor, 66% had headache.*
- Increased intracranial pressure: Usually not excruciating
- Subarachnoid hemorrhage: "Worst headache of my life," with or without transient impairment of consciousness*
- Spontaneous dissection of the internal carotid artery: Present in 70% of cases
- Cerebellar hemorrhage: Headache, vomiting, and inability to walk with normal lower extremity strength*

*From Weiner W, Goetz C, eds: *Neurology for the non-neurologist,* ed 3, Philadelphia, 1993, Lippincott; and Ropper A: *Neurological and neurosurgical intensive care,* ed 3, New York, 1993, Raven.

neurologic problems such as tumors to go undetected because of negative patient history for headache and normal results of neurologic examinations (Becker et al., 1993).

Although triage nurses may feel bad if a patient with a headache whom they have triaged as "nonurgent" or "urgent" turns out to have increased ICP or a brain tumor, it is not realistic to expect to detect all gross abnormalities in triage and the nurse should learn from experience rather than be self-denigrating.

All patients with a headache should be provided with a quiet, dark place to rest, if possible, until they are seen in the ED. An emesis basin should also be provided if they are nauseated or have vomited because of the headache pain.

Emergency departments often see patients with headaches whose primary aim for seeking ED services is to obtain narcotics. The human response to these patients is often frustration and anger in health care providers who have chosen to work in the ED to serve patients with "true" medical or traumatic emergencies. With the upsurge in violence toward health care providers an attitude of discomfort and an unspoken policy to rapidly dismiss the patient—"medicate them and get them out of here"—are also common; although time efficient in the short run, these responses are likely to result in the frequent return of the patient to the ED for similar treatment. An understanding of the process of addiction is helpful in learning how to deal effectively and therapeutically with "drug-seeking" patients. Health care providers must remember that patients are often addicted to prescription drugs because narcotics were prescribed to keep them from being a "nuisance" to health care providers; rather then being provided with a full evaluation of the root of their problem, they were provided with a prescription and dismissed. A team approach to patients with headaches involving mental health personnel, pain specialists, and ED professionals would be helpful in developing a systematic plan for triage and treatment of patients who frequently present themselves to the ED with a chief complaint of headache. To keep from enabling these behaviors and to redirect patients to appropriate treatment options, the ability to keep a record of patients with drug-seeking behaviors is also necessary.

Syncope or Dizziness

Syncope is one of the most difficult symptoms to evaluate. Descriptions by patients of dizziness or a whirring, spinning sensation should be recorded within quotation marks. Orthostatic vital signs and an apical pulse check should be obtained in patients with syncope, to evaluate for signs of hemodynamic instability and cardiac rate and/or rhythm disturbances. Patients with a history of cardiac problems or who are at high risk should be immediately triaged into a monitored bed by wheelchair to avoid the risk of a fall. Other useful assessments may include rapid urine pregnancy testing for women and girls of childbearing age, pulse oximetry, and rapid blood sugar measurement. The cost and duration of the additional procedures enter into the triage nurse's judgment of their immediate relevancy to triage decision making so that such procedures are used prudently.

Any pediatric patient with any of the aforementioned problems should be triaged into the ED immediately, and weight and weight changes must be assessed, since pediatric diabetes is heralded by weight loss and changes in affect and energy level, which are sometimes overlooked, with tragic results.

A chief complaint of syncope or dizziness may be the result of a simple problem such as inadequate food or fluid ingestion, it may be a side effect of nonprescription or prescription medication or combination of medications, or it may be a pathophysiologic problem such as Meniere's disease or a transient

---

BOX 6–9	**Key Questions To Ask Patients With Syncope or Dizziness**

- When did it start?
- What do you think may have brought it on?
- Can you describe how it feels?
- Do you feel dizzy or does the room seem to spin?
- Is it continuous or does it come and go?
- Have you been exposed to any chemicals or cleaning products that you are aware of? If so, describe the ventilation in the area where the exposure took place.
- Have you experienced vomiting, palpitations, or any other symptoms?
- Have you taken nonprescription medications? Are you taking prescription medications?
- When was your last alcoholic drink? When was it taken in relation to any medications?

BOX 6–10	**Risk Factors for Cerebrovascular Accident**

- Oral contraceptives
- Previously undetected hypertension
- Mitral valve prolapse
- Patent foramen ovale with paradoxic embolism
- Hypercoagulation
- Metabolic disorders
- Cocaine abuse (subarachnoid hemorrhage, intracerebral hemorrhage, and cerebral infarction)
- Regular alcohol consumption
- Smoking
- Amphetamine abuse

ischemic attack (TIA). As with all complaints, the triage process begins with a careful history (Box 6–9).

Designation of triage level depends on the potential origins or causes of the patient's syncope and the patient's triage history and physical examination. As with headache, syncope or dizziness may herald a critical neurologic problem. One of the common, critical problems, particularly in older patients, is cerebrovascular accident (CVA); this possibility should also be considered in younger patients who have risk factors for CVA (Box 6–10)

Although syncope may be one symptom of a CVA, there are many other symptoms of this problem. The nurse should consider the possibility that the patient may have any of four types of CVA: thrombotic or embolic infarct, or intracerebral or subarachnoid hemorrhage. With thrombotic CVA a TIA commonly occurs before the full event, and symptoms of this prodrome may include syncope or dizziness, numbness around the lips or face, transient blindness or diplopia, aphasia or slurred speech, and single-extremity sensory and motor difficulties or ataxia (Box 6–11). Furthermore, thrombotic CVAs or TIAs are often nocturnal, and symptoms first become evident on awakening (Weiner and Goetz, 1993).

If the nurse suspects interruption of blood flow to the brain,

BOX 6–11	**Common Signs of a Transient Ischemic Attack**

- Transient blindness or diplopia
- Aphasia or slurred speech
- Single-extremity sensory and motor difficulties
- Ataxia
- Syncope or dizziness
- Numbness around the lips or face

one source of occlusion may be assessed in triage—the carotid arteries. The nurse should palpate for bilateral carotid pulsations, taking care not to massage the carotid sinus, which may cause the patient to have a vasovagal reaction. The triage nurse may listen over the carotid arteries with the bell of the stethoscope for bruits (a whooshing sound caused by turbulent blood flow as a result of blood swirling through an occluded or narrow artery), but patients should be asked to hold their breath momentarily during auscultation to avoid mistaking tracheal breath sounds for bruits. The nurse should also observe the patients for symmetry of the face and ask about symptoms of TIAs.

As mentioned earlier, there are many possible causes for syncope or dizziness, including cardiac dysrhythmias, hypotension, blood loss, Meniere's disease, hypoglycemia, TIAs, and CVAs. If the nurse suspects that the symptom may indicate a critical neurologic or serious medical problem, a thorough, brief physical assessment should be performed, and detected deviations from normal should be entered into the triage record (Box 6–12).

SEIZURES

Triage evaluation of patients with a presenting complaint of having had a seizure is usually brief and direct, since such patients are designated as "emergent" and (ideally) enter the ED quite rapidly. According to Ropper's acute-treatment protocol for seizures, it is crucial to assess cardiorespiratory function, obtain a history, and perform a neurologic and physical exam-

BOX 6–12	**Useful Physical Assessment Techniques for Patients With Syncope or Dizziness**

- Vital signs, including apical pulse
- Orthostatic vital signs, particularly in the patient with persistent dizziness or pallor and dizziness on arising
- Assessment of pupil size, symmetry, and reaction to light
- Observation of the patient's gait for asymmetry, ataxia, or difficulty
- Assessment of hand grip for equality and strength
- Listening to speech for clarity and articulation
- Assessment of language for expression of logical ideas and ability to provide information requiring recall
- Measurement of blood sugar level by Accucheck or one-touch method if available
- Pulse oximetry, if hypoxemia is suspected

ination on the patient and to confirm the diagnosis by observing one seizure or ongoing seizure activity (Ropper, 1993).

When the triage nurse is the first person to observe seizure activity on an incoming patient and ED personnel are not immediately available, the triage nurse brings the patient into the ED and stays with the patient, observing the seizure and supporting the patient's airway while obtaining vital information, if possible, from the family or others accompanying the patient.

Patients who are brought to the ED after having had a seizure at home and who have a history of seizure activity such as epilepsy should be observed for persistent neurologic signs, since "neurologic signs that persist after seizures (even if transient, e.g., Todd's postictal paralysis) suggest an underlying structural brain lesion . . ." (Weisberg et al., 1993). If the results of neurologic examination are normal, the triage nurse may take the time to obtain a careful history for determination of risk factors that may precipitate seizures (Box 6–13). When a drug overdose is suspected or a drug-induced seizure is thought to be possible, a urine screen for toxicologic study should be obtained as soon as possible.

| BOX 6–13 | **Risk Factors That May Precipitate Seizures** |

- Sleep deprivation
- Alcohol overdose or withdrawal from alcohol in chronic-phase alcoholism
- Prescription drugs: Antihistamines, anticholinergics, amphetamines, antidepressants, or antipsychotics
- Illicit drugs: Phencyclidine, marijuana, cocaine, amphetamines, "Ts" and "blues" containing pentazocine (Talwin) and tripelennamine (Pyribenzamine)
- Emotional stress
- Fever
- Diet
- Head trauma
- Hypoglycemia

HEAD AND NECK PROBLEMS
Head Injury

The patient with a chief complaint of head injury, because of the structure involved and the importance of the organ housed within the skull, must take priority for evaluation without delay (Box 6–14). Head injuries that involve minor trauma without loss of consciousness result in "nonurgent" classification. A patient with a report of head injury who is conscious at presentation may be designated as "emergent" if there is concern that brain trauma has occurred or is imminent. As with all other presenting problems, patients should not be evaluated solely on appearance. Critical questions must be asked immediately to ascertain the likelihood of a severe problem or the potential for serious sequelae or complications.

The first priority of the triage nurse is to determine the mechanism of the trauma. A concern for the possibility of spinal trauma is ever present, and if such trauma is at all suspected, the patient should be placed in a cervical collar in supine position and immediately triaged into the ED for care. Other consequences of head trauma that should be considered throughout the course of the history include skull fracture, brain injury,

BOX 6–14	**Critical Findings in Evaluation of Head Injury That Results in Emergent Triage Designation**

- Loss of consciousness for more than 5 minutes
- Major mechanism of injury
- Depressed level of consciousness
- Disorientation
- Speech or language difficulties that are new
- Report of traumatic seizure
- Motor deficits involving movement difficulties or unequal strength
- Pupils that are unequal in size or slow to respond to light
- Fluid or blood drainage from the ears or nose
- "Raccoon" eyes or Battle's sign

mouth or tongue injury, and damage to structures involving the airway. Specific concern for these consequences develops as a result of the history and the patient's physical presentation. In cases of motor vehicle accident the patient's position in the car should be determined, as well as use of seatbelt and whether the patient struck the windshield, was ejected, or struck other objects in the car at the time of impact, such as another person's head (see Chapter 1, Box 1–10). If the patient was injured in a bicycle, motorcycle, or roller-blading accident, the use of a helmet and condition of the helmet, if used, should be ascertained. Patients who have had a fall should be queried about the distance of the fall, the trauma sustained during the fall, and their position on landing, and should be asked whether they walked after the fall.

If the mechanism is penetrating trauma, such as a knife or gunshot wound, the patient is usually triaged immediately for trauma care, but if the patient's condition appears stable, and the triage nurse can begin gathering a history, the type of weapon and distance from the perpetrator should be determined, to help predict the type of injuries the patient has. The nurse should be alert to signs and symptoms of skull fracture, particularly basilar and depressed skull fractures, since linear skull fractures can be detected only by x-ray. Patients who have had a basilar skull fracture may have CSF discharge from the nose or ears or both, tinnitus, facial paralysis, bilateral black eyes or "raccoon" eyes (3 to 4 hours after injury), or bruising behind the ears, that is, Battle's sign (6 to 8 hours after injury). In patients who have a depressed skull fracture, the skull is pressing on the brain from the trauma (Tess and Murphy, 1986). This condition is best evaluated by inspection only; the physician, wearing sterile gloves, then examines the wound more closely in the ED.

Most immediately the patient and, if possible, witnesses to the accident should be asked whether a loss of consciousness occurred after the injury was sustained. If there was a loss of consciousness, the amount of time the patient was unconscious should be estimated as accurately as possible. If the patient is a

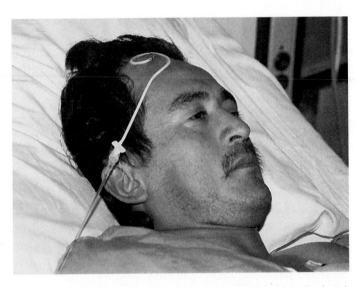

Fig. 6–2 Patients with a history of falling and striking the head, even in a seemingly minor accident, should be questioned about loss of consciousness. This patient suffered a "simple fall" and was found to have increased intracranial pressure.

child, the historian should be asked whether a seizure ensued directly after the child received the injury. As in all injuries, the mechanism of trauma and nature of the sustained injury should be discussed briefly and essential details recorded. Anatomic figures in the chart format, if available, may be used to record the location of the injury. Assessment of a patient with a head injury should be rapid, and care must be taken to avoid stimulating the individual, since overstimulation could increase the patient's risk for elevation of ICP (Jackson, 1992) (Fig. 6–2).

A physical assessment performed in triage on a patient with a reported head injury should focus on the critical elements of a neurologic assessment (Box 6–15).

Evaluation of the patient's orientation should be performed in sequences since it is typical for patients to lose their orientation to time, place, and person, in that order. Start with asking the day and date and progress to asking whether the patient can state the month and year. Any deficit should be recorded specifically. To evaluate the patient correctly, it is important for the examiner to know the right answers to the questions. If the

---

BOX 6–15	**Critical Features in the Assessment of Head Injury**

- Mechanism of injury
- Loss of consciousness
- Current level of consciousness (including orientation to time, place, and person)
- Speech (ability to articulate clearly) and language (ability to express oneself logically)
- Motor function (all extremities moving and showing equal strength)
- Sensory function (ability to perceive touch)
- Pupil equality and response to light
- Fluid or blood drainage from the nose or ears
- Bruising of both eyes or behind ears
- Intact function of cranial nerves I, III, IV, VI, VII, and VIII: Check sense of smell, ability to perform extraocular muscle movements smoothly and symmetrically, ability to perform symmetric facial expressions, and hearing

patient cannot name the location specifically (e.g., General Hospital) but can state that she/he is in a hospital or an ambulance, the patient should be credited with an appropriate response. To be credited, correct identification of the person is necessary.

Assessment of speech and language is done concurrently with the interview, since patients are speaking and expressing themselves in response to the examiner's queries. Problems with articulation of sound, perseverative responses or questions, or illogical or poor thought progression are best documented succinctly, using the patient's exact responses to the examiner's questions. Be sure that questions for which an illogical or disjointed answer is given are rephrased and that the patient understands the question before determining that disorientation exists. Also be sure that sensory organs are functioning normally, that is, that the patient can hear. In the triage setting the patient's gross motor and sensory functions are evaluated. The nurse observes the patient's gait if the patient has ambulated into the facility for care, checks for equal hand grips, and can simply touch the patient over four to six general locations on the upper extremities with the patient's eyes closed, asking the patient to state "now" when the patients feels that she/he is being touched. The stimulus should be scattered but cover the same areas bilaterally, and the rate of the stimulus should be varied so that it will not be predictable and cause the patient to state "now" simply because she/he expects the next touch to occur. Pupils should always be measured with a pupil gauge for accuracy; even slight inequity is critical.

A suspicion that there is fluid drainage from the nose or ears should be investigated and documented for the characteristics of the fluid (consistency, color, amount, and odor). Further evaluation such as assessment of cranial nerves and reflexes may be necessary but is not appropriate in the triage setting because of time constraints. The Glasgow Coma Scale (Chapter 1, Box 1–14) should be employed to objectively document the patient's neurologic state on presentation.

It is critical to remember that all patients with facial trauma should be interviewed and evaluated as head injury patients, in addition to assessment of the specifics of the facial trauma and injuries. The presence of bilateral black eyes (raccoon eyes) or bruising behind the ears (Battle's sign) indicates a need for emergent triage to care, since these may indicate basilar skull fracture.

Head injuries are frightening to patients and their families, and patients with seemingly simple problems such as a "goose egg" on the forehead without a history of loss of consciousness frequently seek medical attention at the ED. Reassurance of patient and family should occur after the triage evaluation. This is necessary in order to establish a relationship with the patient and facilitate compliance with the designated level of triage, if less than emergent.

Furthermore, in the head-injured child, slowly developing cerebral edema can go relatively unnoticed for the first 6 to 18 hours, and the parents may need to be informed about the necessity for careful reassessment of the child, even if he/she is eventually discharged from the ED. Clinical approaches that keep the child calm (and the ICP down) during assessments are important in triage (Patterson et al., 1992).

Sometimes children who suffer a simple fall may sustain critical neurologic trauma that is not immediately evident on presentation for medical care in those who are alert and have normal vital signs. In a review of 53 children with a diagnosis of traumatic epidural hematoma at Boston Children's Hospital between 1980 and 1990, an epidural hematoma developed in 24 of the children after a fall of less than 5 feet. At the time of diagnosis, 51 of 53 children had one or more symptoms of vomiting, headache, or lethargy. Twenty-six patients were alert, 21 were responsive to verbal or painful stimuli, and only 5 were unresponsive or posturing. Twenty-one patients had acute neurologic deterioration before surgery; however, 20 were alert and had normal vital signs and neurologic examination results at diagnosis. Loss of consciousness at the time of head injury was not an accurate predictor of neurologic trauma, since posttraumatic loss of consciousness occurred in only 10 of the patients (duration of the loss was more than 5 minutes in only 3), was unknown in 12 patients, and did not occur in 31 patients. Thirty-six of the 53 children had skull fractures. "The majority of children had normal vital signs, normal pupillary size and reactivity, nonfocal neurologic examination, and normal LOC with each sign considered independently" (Schultzman et al., 1993).

Epidural hematomas are critical neurologic events and may

be difficult to suspect because, even in patients who have had a loss of consciousness, a ''lucid interval'' of hours may cause the patient, health care providers, and family to think that the patient is normal. An awareness of this danger is helpful in impressing on family, even at the outset of triage, which signs are important to watch for and report, should they be observed. Patients in whom an epidural hematoma develops usually have received blunt trauma to the temporal or temporoparietal region, which causes a laceration of the meningeal blood vessels and consequent accumulation of blood between the dura and skull. If the epidural hematoma is not recognized and promptly evacuated by means of neurosurgery, brain herniation and death may ensue (Robinson, 1994).

Treatment of patients with a head injury in the triage area is limited but useful. Offering an ice pack and, if possible, a quiet environment is also helpful for patient comfort. Furthermore, efforts to control bleeding and other consequences of head trauma help minimize the effects of the injury and provide patient comfort until the patient is seen in the ED (Box 6–16).

Any child with a head injury who may have been the victim of abuse should immediately be referred for a social service evaluation when available so that reporting to child protective services is accomplished. In the absence of available social services personnel, the suspected abuse should be directly reported by the nurse to the appropriate agency (social services or law enforcement). Agencies should immediately be notified whenever there is a concern that the child cannot or should not be sent home because she/he might not be safe at home. Referrals to public health agencies should be initiated within the ED whenever safety concerns arise, to provide a safety check of the

BOX 6–16	**Triage Treatment of Patients With Head Injury**

- Airway support
- Cervical collar and spinal support
- Control of bleeding with direct pressure and temporary dressing
- Ice (as appropriate)

home environment and patient teaching regarding injury and accident prevention by public health nurses.

Hallucinations and Problems With Orientation and Memory

Patients or family members of patients who have a chief complaint of hallucination or problems with orientation or memory, or both, must be interviewed thoroughly. The triage nurse must be careful not to assume that the patient's complaints are related to mental health, since any of these presentations have potential neurologic, endocrine, and circulation causes or may be related to effects of prescription drugs, nonprescription medications, or intake of alcohol or street drugs.

Patients complaining of hallucinations must be asked about the nature of the hallucinations (visual, olfactory, auditory, and so forth) and their specific content. For example, a patient who is having auditory hallucinations such as voices should be asked to describe the voices and what they are saying. Impulse control should also be evaluated to determine whether these patients are a potential threat to themselves or others, so they can be triaged accordingly. It should also be determined whether the patient has a chronic mental health problem such as schizophrenia; if so, compliance with pharmacologic therapy should be investigated. Many schizophrenics have insight into the degree of their psychosis and will honestly appraise the degree of danger they feel. Others with schizophrenia may have a paranoid component to their illness, and if they pose a hazard to themselves or others, immediate involuntary restraint may be necessary.

In patients with a chief complaint relating to orientation or memory loss or both, immediate focus on the time and manner of onset should occur. The patient deserves immediate or emergent triage into the ED if neuroendocrine problems are suspected. In patients who have a history of diabetes a rapid blood sugar level may be obtained, and appropriate treatment such as is possible in the triage area should ensue if the ED cannot handle the patient in a timely fashion. Patients with hyperglycemia may be provided with plenty of water to drink, and those with hypoglycemia should be given 4 ounces of juice and crackers.

When the patient's level of orientation is the specific concern, the patient should be specifically asked to tell the triage nurse the day, date, month, and year (time); the specific name of the facility or type of facility where the patient currently is (place); and person and self, since this is the order in which orientation is usually lost. Use of the patient's exact words is helpful in recording succinctly the patient's condition. Memory can be evaluated surreptitiously during demographic data gathering and with general questions such as "Are you allergic to any medications?" Although the reliability of the informant is impaired by the present complaint and the patient's answers should be validated by a secondary source, the responses may be a clue to the degree of impairment and the patient's insight regarding the problem.

Attention should be paid to the patient's speech and language, and deviations described succinctly. Speech problems that may be evident include problems with articulation of sounds that form words. Problems with language may include problems with word selection, circumlocution, perseveration (repeating words or phrases often), or difficulty maintaining train of thought.

Problems with mental status are alarming and frightening to patients and family members. The triage nurse can help by providing reassurance and clarifying what will happen next. The use of volunteers to keep families apprised of when they might be seen and to ensure that they know where their basic needs may be met is especially helpful.

Vision Disturbance

Although vision disturbance is being discussed as a neurologic problem, it is important, of course, to realize that vision disturbances such as diplopia or blurred vision may be a result of eye trauma or a foreign body in the eye. However, problems with vision may cue the examiner to a problem in the occipital lobe of the brain, a problem with the optic cranial nerve, retinal problems, or problems with other systems such as the endocrine system. Patients who enter triage with a vague complaint such as "I'm having difficulty seeing" should be interviewed in detail (Box 6–17). They should be asked whether the change is acute or has been noticed over time, and should be queried about precipitating factors, the medical history, and usual visual acuity and whether corrective lenses (if so, what type) were

---

| BOX 6–17 | **Evaluation of Vision Disturbance** |

- Inquire about onset of the problem (acute or gradual)
- Ask about precipitants to the symptom (exposure to toxic fumes or fluids, head injury, and so forth)
- Assess the appearance of both eyes, and record findings (infection, discharge, foreign bodies, or lack of obvious signs of problems)
- Assess visual acuity: Central vision (near and far) and peripheral vision

---

used. Cleaning solutions (brand and type) that have been used to treat contacts and frequency of cleaning should be investigated. Visual acuity should be evaluated for distant, near, and peripheral vision. Patients complaining about halos around lights should be asked specifically whether they are on a regimen of digitalis; if the answer is affirmative, toxic effects of digitalis should be suspected and a measurement of digitalis levels should be ordered.

If there is a suspicion that toxins—whether fluid or fumes—have affected the patient's vision, the patient should be treated immediately and the eyes lavaged (Fig. 6–3). When a foreign body is in the eyes, proparacaine hydrochloride or another, similar ophthalmic anesthetic may be applied to decrease the patient's pain during waiting. Standard medical orders should be in place for triage nurses to legally administer eye anesthetics. An eye patch, if deemed appropriate, may also be used during the waiting period (Box 6–18).

Eye Injury

Eye injuries are most often minor and most frequently occur when a foreign body to the eye either causes or places the patient at risk for corneal injury or abrasion. Direct trauma to the eye from blunt or sharp force can result in critical injuries to the organ and deserves immediate attention. Arc burns from unprotected exposure to welding flames may also result in an immediate need for treatment. Chemical splash into the eyes that has not been resolved by continuous washing at the site of

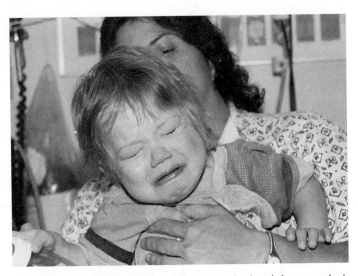

Fig. 6–3 Infants and small children are at high risk for eye splash because they are highly active. Lice shampoo splashed in the eyes is very painful and requires immediate lavage.

the splash may be designated as an emergent condition, to ensure rapid initiation of further lavage of the eyes.

The eyes are a critical sensory organ, and although not every patient with a chief complaint related to the eyes warrants an emergent triage designation, a systematic, rapid evaluation of the condition of the organ and likelihood of morbidity must take place. Of primary importance is a clear history of the eye insult (Box 6–19). If a blunt injury occurred, such as a tennis ball hitting the eye, the patient should be asked whether protective eyewear was used and asked to estimate the possible velocity of the ball and the angle at which the ball hit the eye. If a sharp injury occurred, such as an arrow hitting the eye, the condition obviously must be triaged into the ED as emergent, but the material and length of the arrow should still be determined, to aid in treatment planning. If the patient reports unprotected exposure to welding light, the eyes should be immediately patched and examination should occur as quickly as possible, to determine the extent of injury. A report of chemical splash to the eyes necessitates inquiry to determine the com-

| BOX 6–18 | **Vision Treatments That May be Ordered or Initiated in Triage** |

- Lavage
- Ophthalmic anesthetization
- Eye patch
- Rapid measurement of glucose level, if glycemic abnormalities are suspected

| BOX 6–19 | **Critical Questions in History of Injury or Insult to the Eye** |

BLUNT TRAUMA

Object causing injury, velocity of force, direction of force onto eye

SHARP TRAUMA

Object size and composition, velocity of force, direction of force onto eye

ARC BURN

Distance from flame, duration of exposure, time since exposure

CHEMICAL SPLASH

Chemical name(s), irrigation substance and duration of irrigation, initial eye symptoms and current symptoms

pound or exact chemical that has been splashed and whether treatment (eye rinsing) ensued immediately after the splash or was instituted at all. Any insult to the eyes may have systemic consequences, so it is appropriate to call a poison control center, to report the incident, to investigate particular consequences of exposure to a specified chemical, and to define the most appropriate therapy.

Physical evaluation of the eyes in the triage setting (briefly

BOX 6–20	Rapid Eye Assessment

- Direct eye assessment for inflammation, trauma, and presence of foreign bodies
- Vision testing
- Extraocular movement testing
- Determination of eye pH

summarized in Box 6–20) includes direct inspection of the eye for signs of inflammation, photophobia, and the presence of obvious foreign bodies (using a penlight to examine the cornea with tangential and direct lighting); assessment of pupil size, equality, and direct and consensual response to light; testing for intact extraocular muscles by means of the extraocular movement (EOM) test; and testing of central near and distant vision and peripheral vision. Signs of inflammation for which the eyes should be assessed include pain, redness (usually erythema of palpebral conjunctiva or infection of the sclera), edema (periorbital, palpebral or bulbar conjunctiva, or edema of the sclera), warmth (periorbital, such as might be evident in cellulitis), and loss of function (evaluated by assessment of vision and EOMs and patient report of specific eye difficulty). Pupil size must be assessed with a pupil-measuring instrument or pupil eye card, not estimated by the triage nurse by means of visual inspection (Fig. 6–4). Even minor deviations may be critical and should be reported.

If photophobia or obvious eye sensitivity exists, it is advisable to protect the patient's eyes from light until the examination and treatment occur. Protection may include having the patient put on dark glasses or double patching the eyes. If a chemical splash has occurred, these initial, temporary treatments are deferred, since the most appropriate action is to institute immediate eye lavage. Immediately before eye lavage it may be useful to determine the pH of the eye by using a reagent strip. This information may be helpful in determining the type of chemical and ensuing consequences, particularly when the

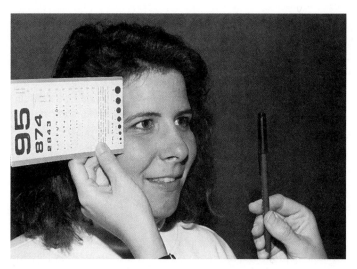

Fig. 6–4 Pupil assessment requires a pupil gauge for accuracy. Pupils should be assessed for size and symmetry.

patient cannot name the chemical to which the eyes have been exposed. Poison control centers should be able to provide advice on specific chemicals and appropriate treatment. Response of the pupils to light is assessed by shining a light directly into each pupil and watching for constriction with light (direct) and by watching the opposite pupil when the light is shone directly into a pupil (consensual).

Many nurses and health care providers record the mnemonic PERRLA for pupil assessment. PERRL may be a concise form of charting if, indeed, the examiner has determined that the *p*upils are *e*qual (recording size), *r*ound, and *r*eactive (direct and consensual) to *l*ight. Most often the *A* of this acronym has not been evaluated. The *A* stands for *a*ccommodation and indicates that the examiner has assessed the pupil for constriction when the patient looks at a near object and dilation when the patient looks at a distant object. Some examiners integrate assessment for accommodation by watching the pupil when the eyes converge at the end of EOM testing by having the patient observe the examiner's finger as it moves toward the patient's nose. However, this is not a critical eye assessment in triage and can be omitted.

Assessment of the extraocular muscles gives the examiner information regarding the intact state of cranial nerves III, IV, and VI. The extraocular movement (EOM) test is useful in determining the effects of an injury on both the muscles and the cranial nerves that operate the eyes. The most rapid way of testing EOMs is to perform the H test; the examiner must realize that it is best to progress slowly through the six cardinal fields of gaze. The examiner observes the patient's eyes to see that the movement of the eyes is smooth and symmetric (Fig. 6–5). In addition, during the performance of the EOMs the examiner may observe the patient's eyes for the presence of nystagmus (rapid oscillation of the eyes in the lateral fields), which may indicate cerebellar dysfunction. This would be most appropriate in the patient with eye injury who sustained facial trauma and who may also have a brain injury.

Central vision testing should usually be performed in the ED using a Snellen chart (Fig. 6–6, *A*) but central vision may

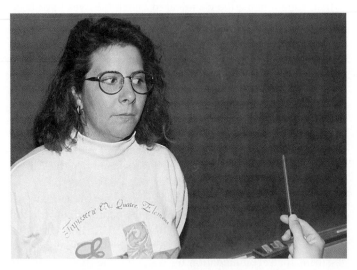

Fig. 6–5 When testing extraocular movement, the examiner watches the patient's eyes to see that they move smoothly and symmetrically.

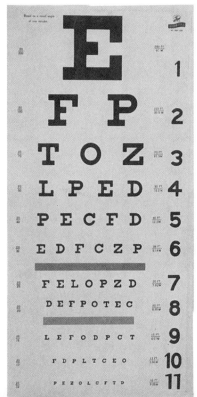

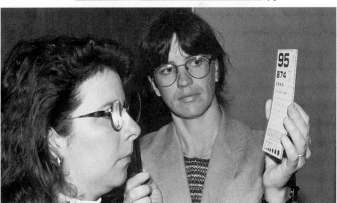

Fig. 6–6 **A,** The Snellen chart should be at eye level in a well-lit area for accurate assessment of distant visual acuity. **B,** A Rosenbaum hand-held eye vision card can be used for testing central vision also.

be assessed initially if the triage nurse has a hand-held Rosenbaum card and printed material to check for acuity of distant and near vision (Fig. 6–6, *B*). The patient with corrective lenses should wear them, since the assessment is not a complete eye examination but an evaluation for changes from the patient's corrected, normal vision. Peripheral vision can be tested using a confrontation test to check for gross loss of peripheral vision. If the patient is wearing contact lenses, they should be removed as quickly and gently as possible to prevent further potential trauma to the cornea.

Direct examination of the eyes for the presence of foreign bodies may be difficult because of the eye discomfort felt by the patient. Instillation of an eye anesthetic such as proparacaine in the triage area (with standing orders) gives pain relief to the patient while allowing for direct examination of the cornea. Observation for foreign bodies should be done by looking directly and from the side into the eye, using direct and tangential lighting to illuminate flecks that may otherwise be indistinguishable. Gross assessment is helpful but does not replace examination of the eye with a slit lamp in the ED.

The patient with obvious eye trauma resulting in hyphema (blood in the anterior chamber) or damage to the globe requires immediate evaluation. In the interim period eye patching should be gentle but secure.

Patients with eye injury must always be asked about tetanus status, and their risk for infection should always be considered. A brief list of eye treatments is given in Box 6–21. When eye trauma has been a result of domestic violence or child abuse, the examiner must notify the proper authorities and ini-

---

BOX 6–21	**Eye Treatments**

- Irrigation
- Eye patch
- Tetanus booster
- Ophthalmic anesthetic

---

tiate paperwork that enters the victim into the appropriate social service and law enforcement systems.

Ear Pain

The most frequent cause of ear pain is otitis media. The pattern of the presenting illness—rhinorrhea, severe ear pain, and often fever—makes it easy to determine. The patient, although in great discomfort, can usually be triaged as ''nonurgent'' or ''urgent,'' since the complaint is not life threatening. The triage nurse must be aware, of course, that although ear pain is most often related to infection or inflammation, such as in otitis externa, other causes cannot be ruled out and it should not be instantly assumed that the patient with ear pain has otitis. Parents and child-care providers with pediatric patients complaining of ear pain should be asked whether the children (particularly those who are too young to answer clearly for themselves) have been pulling at their ears or whether it is suspected that they might have put something into the ear. After the history is taken, the external ear should be examined for the presence of discharge or obvious foreign bodies. Treatment of pain and/or fever with weight-based dosage of acetaminophen should be initiated if the patient is not allergic to acetaminophen, has not been adequately dosed at home, and has not received a dose of acetaminophen within a time frame that prevents a repeat dose of the medication. If the child is wrapped too warmly, excess clothing should be removed.

When patients enter the ED with a chief complaint of a live insect in the ear, it is important that the patient be triaged or treated immediately because of the severe discomfort and distress the insect causes. Insects that are found in the ear include common houseflies, cockroaches, and earwigs. Shining a light directly into the ear may cause the insect to exit the canal as it follows the light. If this treatment is not immediately successful, mineral oil should be instilled into the canal to drown the insect and decrease the irritation felt by the patient as the insect frantically tries to exit the canal. Once the insect is removed or drowned, the patient may wait for the examination with a triage designation of urgent. Patients with foreign bodies in the ear that do not cause severe discomfort or threaten the integrity of the ear can be triaged as ''nonurgent'' or ''urgent'' depending on agency policy. Safety education regarding size-appropriate toys and food for children under 3 years of age who have inserted such items as beads or peanuts into their ears may begin in the triage area. Children who have soft items such as bread in the ear sometimes insert these items into the canal to ease ear pain resulting from otitis media. Irrigation of the canal is not recommended, since bread absorbs the water and swells, thereby becoming more difficult to remove. Irrigation of the ear canal is not advised when otitis media and perforation of the tympanic membrane are possible.

Occasionally patients may have ear drainage that does not occur as a result of a ruptured tympanic membrane but is a result of CSF leak. This leak is most often associated with head trauma, particularly injury to the parietal skull. Any suspected CSF leak should be triaged as emergent. Testing the fluid for glucose level and checking it for halo can be used as early determinations of the presence of CSF or ear discharge resulting from a tympanic membrane rupture.

Dental Emergencies

Patients who arrive at the triage area with a chief complaint related to the teeth come to the ED because they do not have a dentist or know of a dental clinic they can go to for urgent care or because they have injuries or problems that also involve the face.

When a patient complains of toothache, it should be determined whether the patient has a dentist, funds for seeing a dentist, or dental insurance that may make it possible to triage the patient directly to dental service. Patients who do not have access to dental services are most likely to be triaged as ''nonurgent'' or ''urgent'' depending on the degree of discomfort, the ability of the ED to handle the patient in a timely fashion, and the presence of other symptoms such as fever. As with any patient with discomfort or fever, weight-appropriate acetaminophen treatment can be initiated in triage. The cervical and tonsillar lymph nodes of patients with fever should be palpated, and characteristics of enlarged nodes—size, consistency, location, mobility, and tenderness—recorded.

Patients who have traumatic dislodgment of a tooth are often distressed, since this most frequently occurs with central

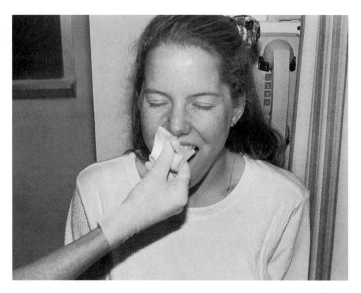

Fig. 6–7 Pressure using a 4 × 4 pad can be applied to replace a dislodged tooth.

and lateral incisors, with obvious cosmetic consequence. If the patient does not arrive with the dislodged tooth and the accident has occurred within 1 hour, the patient's family or anyone who may locate the tooth should be solicited to do so, and to store it in milk or sterile water. If the patient arrives with an intact tooth, it should be rinsed with sterile water and reinserted as quickly as possible, then held with pressure by the patient or a person accompanying the patient until it is secured in place by an oral surgeon or dentist (Fig. 6–7).

Lice

Patients who complain of severe itching of the scalp or occipital lymph node enlargement, or both, should be suspected of having pediculosis or head lice. The triage nurse may be able to verify the presence of lice by donning gloves and examining the scalp and hair follicles for lice and nits. If time does not permit the triage nurse to examine the patient, the patient may be triaged out when possible for service at a clinic or a private medical office. Patients who must be seen in the ED should be isolated until they can be evaluated. Some patients have concerns regarding treatment such as a worry about eye irritation resulting from lice shampoo eye splash. Determining who arrived at the diagnosis of lice is important, since many people unnecessarily treat the condition before the diagnosis has been verified and others overtreat it. When the triage nurse is able to advise the patient without medical examination (in obvious cases of head lice), permethrin or pyrethrins should be recommended because it is available without prescription and is most effective in eradicating pediculosis. In triage referral for pharmacy treatment, complete instructions regarding lice treatment should also be provided. Patients should always be cautioned about overtreatment, since lice shampoo in excess may have neurotoxic effects that can cause seizures and death.

Facial Emergencies

Patients with facial trauma are of twofold concern to the triage nurse. The primary concern is that any patient with facial trauma may also have brain trauma. Whether the patient lost consciousness and, if so, the duration of unconsciousness at the time of the injury should be determined immediately. If the loss of consciousness was more than momentary, collaboration with the charge nurse should ensue. The patient is usually triaged as ''emergent'' and, depending on the mechanism of injury and the patient's history at presentation and a brief physical examination, the patient may be designated as a trauma patient (Box 6–22).

The second concern of the triage nurse is to evaluate the tissue trauma and initiate measures to control bleeding and minimize swelling. Attention to tetanus status should not be overlooked. Careful examination of sensory organs, particularly the eyes, should occur. Rapid examination of the mouth to evaluate dental and oral tissue trauma is necessary. When the patient is bleeding profusely and is under the influence of alcohol or street drugs, the triage nurse should take precautions to protect against blood spatter and the examiner should be careful when putting her/his fingers into the patient's mouth. Universal precautions are advised in all situations, but a plastic hood and gown may be necessary when the risk of contamination is heightened.

Patients with facial trauma who have lost facial tissue are often candidates for plastic surgery and reattachment. If reattachment of a severed part is possible, the tissue, for example, the lip or ear, should be sought and properly stored until the surgery is possible.

If the patient does not have emergent status but is distressed about the extent of the injuries, the wounds should be cleansed as well as possible and dressed to control bleeding. The secondary benefit of applying a temporary dressing is to obscure the injuries from well-meaning others who often increase the patient's anxiety by telling the patient how awful she/he looks. Significant others should be instructed to focus on diversionary conversation instead of increasing the patient's anxiety level.

In addition to evaluation of the patient's tissue trauma and neurovascular status, a quick check of cranial nerve VII (facial) provides information regarding the neurologic integrity of this cranial nerve and the facial muscles it innervates. The patient is asked to perform several facial expressions—smile, frown, and raise eyebrows—while the nurse watches to see that the movements are executed in a smooth, symmetric manner.

Other cranial nerves that warrant the evaluator's attention include nerves III (oculomotor), IV (abducens), and VI (trochlear); these are checked by testing EOMs, as described in the Eye Injury section. Cranial nerves II (optic) and III (oculomotor) may also be assessed by checking the patient's pupils. All other cranial nerves require assessment that is easier to perform, and valid information regarding these nerves is received during the examination in the ED.

BOX 6–22	**Elements of Rapid Neurologic Assessment**

- Level of consciousness
- Speech and language
- Motor function
- Sensory function
- Reflexes (usually not evaluated in triage)

BOX 6–23	Elements of a Comprehensive Neurologic Assessment

- Mental status
- Cranial nerves
- Motor function, including gait
- Sensory function
- Reflexes
- Balance and coordination

As with all traumatic injuries, when violence is the cause of the injuries, the triage nurse must remember to notify appropriate agency personnel.

One facial emergency that deserves mention and varies from facial trauma (although it is sometimes consequential to trauma) is facial paralysis. This problem is often caused by Bell's palsy but may also be the sign of CVA or TIA. A brief neurologic assessment is warranted in patients who are likely to have Bell's palsy and have an urgent triage designation and in patients who may be having an acute neurologic event and have an emergent triage designation (Box 6–23).

REFERENCES

Becker LA et al.: Detection of intracranial tumors, subarachnoid hemorrhages, and subdural hematomas in primary care patients: a report from ASPN, *J Fam Pract* 37(2):135, 1993.

Choi C: Bacterial meningitis, *Clin Geriatr Med* 8(4):889, 1992.

Coderre C: Meningitis: dangers when the diagnosis is viral, *RN* p. 50, August 1989.

Donner C: Subdural hematoma, *Am J Nurs* 93(10):54, 1993.

Jackson S: Assessing a head injury, *Nursing* 22(9):49, 1992.

Jenkins TL: Fulminant meningococcemia in pediatric patients: nursing considerations, *Pediatr Nurs* 18(6):629, 1992.

Patterson R et al: Head injury in the conscious child, *Am J Nurs* p. 22, 1992.

Robinson K: Early signs of epidural hematoma, *J Emerg Nurs* p. 37, April 1994.

Ropper A: *Neurological and neurosurgical intensive care,* ed 3, New York, 1993, Raven.

Schultzman SA et al: Epidural hematomas in children, *Ann Emerg Med* 22(3):535, 1993.

Tess J, Murphy S: *The multi-trauma victim,* Colorado, 1986, Contemporary Learning.

Weiner W, Goetz C, eds: *Neurology for the non-neurologist,* ed 3, Philadelphia, 1993, Lippincott.

Weisberg L, Strub R, Garcia C: *Decision making in adult neurology,* ed 2, 1993, BC Decker.

Weiss J: Assessment and management of the client with headaches, *Nurse Practitioner* 18(4):44, 47, 51–54, 57, 1993.

RECOMMENDED READING

Adams R, Victor M: *Principles of neurology,* ed 5, New York, 1993, McGraw-Hill.

Andersen, G: How to assess the older mind, *RN* p. 34, July 1992.

Barker E, Moore K: Perfecting the art: neurological assessment, *RN* p. 28, April 1992.

Burns KR, Snyder M: Neurological assessment: adaptations for special populations with mental retardation, *J Neurosci Nurs* 23(2):107, 1991.

Hearer A: *DeJong's The neurologic examination,* ed 5, Philadelphia, 1992.

Jackson S: Assessing a head injury, *Nursing* 22(9):49, 1992.

Lower J: Rapid neuro assessment, *Am Nurs* 92(6):38, 1992.

McDonnell Cooke D: Shielding your patient from digitalis toxicity, *Nursing* 22(7):44, 1992.

Saper J et al: *Handbook of headache management,* Baltimore, 1993, Williams & Wilkins.

Walsh-Kelly C et al: Clinical predictors of bacterial versus aseptic meningitis in childhood, *Ann Emerg Med* 21(8):910, 1992.

7 | Thoracic, Cardiac, and Respiratory Problems

For problems involving the thorax, a rapid evaluation is required to determine the status of the patient's respiratory (Box 7–1) and cardiac systems and the structures that support the vital anatomy housed within the thorax. Patients who have complaints involving the thorax often have good cause for concern, since homeostasis of respiratory and cardiac functions is required to maintain life. As in every situation in which the triage nurse is met by a patient who is distressed, a calm manner and reassurance while providing care help to allay the patient's fears in many instances. When the patient needs to be evaluated in the emergency department (ED) but care is delayed, the patient should be encouraged to communicate any changes in symptoms to the triage nurse during the waiting period.

CARDIAC PROBLEMS
Chest Pain

Patients with chest pain receive a rapid assessment of acuity and potential for complications when they first present themselves to the triage professional. There are myriad reasons for chest pain (Box 7–2). Patients who appear to be in acute distress as a result of severe pain, oxygenation compromise, or trauma are seen immediately, since they usually have a need for emergent care. It is important for triage nurses to understand the most common causes and patterns of chest pain, to raise their index of suspicion for various diagnoses.

Based on the patient's pain pattern and specific risk factors for problems involving the thorax, the triage professional makes the most appropriate triage designation. Judgments that are not based on scientific principles but are a result of an assumption that the patient is not having a "real" problem should be

---

BOX 7–1	**Causes of Respiratory Difficulty**

- Obstructed airway
- Known or new-onset respiratory disease (emphysema, asthma, or pneumonia)
- Inhalation of smoke or other toxins
- Narcotics that have a respiratory depressive effect
- Trauma
- Spontaneous crises (e.g., pneumothorax or pleural effusion)
- Fluid overload (e.g., congestive heart failure)

---

avoided through use of the systematic triage assessment approach. It is critical that patients be questioned about a history of prior incidents of the same discomfort, and they should be asked whether prior episodes have been evaluated by a health care professional. Obtaining information about the diagnosis and treatment of problems associated with the thorax is important for patients who are under medical management. This does not mean that the patient will not have a ''fresh'' evaluation and treatment approach at the time of triage, but it is important to remember that patients with previously diagnosed illnesses or a history of injuries to the thorax are more likely to have recurring episodes of the same problem, complications, or sequelae relevant to the disorders already diagnosed. However, if the patient has a history of noncardiac chest pain, for example, panic disorder, the triage nurse should not assume that the current complaint is noncardiac. The assessment should always err in the direction of detail rather than brevity, and the triage nurse should maintain an open mind with all patients, regardless of their history.

Two of the most common causes of chest pain are cardiac disease and anxiety. Although their origins differ greatly, the effects of distress—continuance of chest pain, release of adrenaline, potentially compromised ventilation and oxygenation, and associated symptoms of nausea, vomiting, and diaphoresis—are similar in both groups of patients. The triage professional's response to patients with chest pain is crucial in

BOX 7–2	Common Causes of Chest Pain and Triage Cues

ANEURYSM

Searing, continuous, severe chest pain, often radiating to back, neck, and shoulder; patient may be hypotensive, diaphoretic, syncopal

ANGINA

Pressure or squeezing chest pain, often relieved by rest or nitroglycerin; may be persistent but is usually 20 minutes in duration (unless unstable angina); may occur with sex, activity, anxiety, or after a heavy meal, activity or smoking in cold weather, or at rest; dyspnea, nausea, vomiting, diaphoresis may accompany, as may symptoms of indigestion

ANXIETY

Stabbing or aching chest pain; may last from minutes to hours; associated with anxiety, stressful event, although may occur at rest; hyperventilation (and associated symptoms such as carpal spasms), palpitations, weakness, fear, or sense of impending doom may also be present

COSTOCHONDRITIS

Sharp, severe pain, often localized to affected area with tenderness on palpation; may radiate

MYOCARDIAL INFARCTION

Aching, pressure, squeezing; pain may be severe, radiate to jaw, neck, back; in some patients (especially diabetics with neuropathy) there may be only a vague sense of discomfort; may have pallor or ashen skin, diaphoresis, dyspnea, nausea, vomiting

MUSCLE STRAIN

Aching, may be severe; associated with increased effort, exercise involving the thorax

NOXIOUS FUMES OR SMOKE INHALATION

Searing lung pain or sense of suffocation; generalized burning or pressure associated with dyspnea, hypoxia, cough; history of exposure to fire, pesticides, carbon monoxide leak or intentional exposure aborted, paint, occupational chemical exposure in an

BOX 7–2	**Common Causes of Chest Pain and Triage Cues—cont'd**

unventilated or underventilated area; generalized over entire chest; pallor, ashen skin, cyanosis may be evident

PERICARDITIS

Sharp pain may radiate to shoulder or neck, may be severe, continuous, increased with lying on left side; may have history of recent cardiac surgery, myocardial infarction, or viral illness

PLEURAL PAIN

Sharp, often severe pain; continuous, increased with breathing, coughing or movement; more common in smokers

PNEUMONIA

Severe, general thorax or ''lung'' pain, continuous; accompanied by fever (not always), tachycardia, malaise, cough

PNEUMOTHORAX

Severe, generalized chest pain with sudden onset and associated with acute shortness of breath

PULMONARY EMBOLISM

Severe, sudden onset with acute shortness of breath, positive risk factors such as history of recent long bone fracture

RIB FRACTURE

Severe, localized pain; associated with trauma, osteoporosis, or metastatic cancer; may be accompanied by dyspnea; tenderness over affected area

TACHYDYSRHYTHMIAS

Severe, crushing, generalized pain over chest associated with anxiety, sense of impending doom, and tachycardia

ULCER

Burning or pressure in epigastrium; may radiate across chest

VIRAL ILLNESS

Generalized aching; may be associated with nausea, vomiting, or cough moderating, when possible, the patient's symptoms. The manner of the triage professional should be calm, deliberate, efficient, and concerned. Immediate comfort measures, such as providing an emesis basin or securing a chair for the patient to sit on and a cool cloth for the face, are simple but helpful nursing measures, particularly when the patient may have to wait in the waiting area outside the ED.

When patients are on a regimen of cardiac medications, their compliance and correct use of the medications should be assessed. For example, if a patient with a history of angina arrives at triage with chest pain and has taken three sublingual nitroglycerin tablets, the patient should be asked how old the nitroglycerin is, when the supply was opened, and how it was used. Patients with a history of angina may have an episode of chest pain unrelieved by three subsequent nitroglycerin tablets because the nitroglycerin is crumbled, frequently air exposed, or too old to be effective. If the triage nurse ascertains this information, it should be recorded on the patient's chart and the patient should be taught about the appropriate use of nitroglycerin or other relevant medications. This teaching can be presented in an abbreviated format—but not in a scolding manner—because it is helpful to begin teaching by providing simple information at this time. When a patient perceives a risk related to the history of cardiac disease and medication usage, a necessary ingredient for compliance with therapeutic regimens exists and should be capitalized on.

Using the format given for analysis of a symptom, the patient should be interviewed about the pattern of pain (Box 7–3). Because of the anxiety so often present in patients with chest pain and the potential seriousness of the patient's problem, it may be necessary to perform the limited triage physical assessment concurrently. When questioning patients about chest pain, it is ideal to ask the questions in an open-ended format, taking care not to put words in the patient's mouth in an effort to be efficient. Patients may require closed-ended questions if they are unable to comprehend what information the examiner is seeking by asking the open-ended questions. Examples of what the examiner wants to know may also be helpful in eliciting specific information. A visual analog or numeric scale may be a useful adjunct in determining the severity of pain, particularly

| BOX 7–3 | **Key Questions for Patients With Chest Pain** |

- When did your chest pain start?
- How did the chest pain come on? Was it sudden or gradual? Was it severe immediately or did it worsen with time?
- What were you doing at the time it started?
- What do you think may have caused your chest pain? (If necessary, ask about activity, exposure to chemical fumes, recent traumatic injury, recent surgeries, and stress.)
- How does it feel right now? (Is it squeezing, sharp, dull, or aching?)
- On a scale of 1 to 10, with 10 being the worst pain you've ever felt or imagined, where would you rate your pain at this moment?
- Can you show me where you feel the pain?
- Do you feel it anywhere else (in the flank, epigastrium, arms, neck, or jaw)?
- Do you have any other symptoms (nausea, vomiting, sweatiness, dizziness, or palpitations)?
- Have you done anything to try to make the pain go away, including using any home remedies or nonprescription medications or prescribed medications? If the answer is yes, was it effective? (If patient takes cardiac medications, ask about the age of the medications and compliance with therapeutic regimens, including activity limitations and use of alcohol.)
- Do you have a history of chest pain? Have you ever seen a doctor for this type of pain? Related to this symptom, what has the diagnosis been in the past?
- What made you feel that you should be evaluated for the chest pain today?

when there is a language barrier between patient and provider or if the patient is a child or developmentally disabled (Fig. 7–1). In communities with a large number of deaf persons, signs commonly used to communicate pain should be posted for the health care provider's information. If the patient indicates that she/he has had chest pain for days or weeks, it is important to establish what (finally) brought the patient to the ED. For example, was it an increase in the severity of the pain, worry about

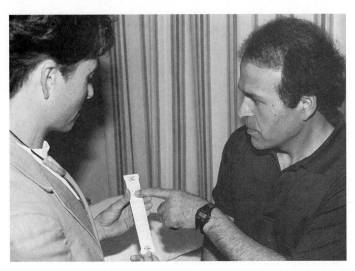

Fig. 7–1   Using a pain scale with a visual aid is especially helpful if a language barrier exists.

the possible reason for the chest pain, associated symptoms that developed or worsened, or encouragement from a concerned significant other? This information is important because it gives the interviewer an immediate understanding of the current state of the patient's symptoms, and it also provides a window to understanding the patient's worst fears and perceptions of the problem. This understanding allows the triage provider to establish a relationship of trust that, it is hoped, will be generalized to the other health care providers with whom the patient will have contact. It also allows the triage professional to tell the patient what will take place following triage and thereby allay any fears associated with the "complete" unknown.

In patients with previously diagnosed illnesses associated with chest pain it is important to learn whether they have contacted their primary health care provider, and this information should be indicated on the record.

As a routine part of the general history taking in triage or when the triage nurse is intuitively concerned that illegal drug use may be a causative factor for chest pain, the patient must

---

BOX 7–4	**Physical Assessment of Patients With Chest Pain**

- Observe skin for diaphoresis, skin color abnormalities, ecchymoses
- Assess airway patency and respiratory pattern
- Assess symmetry and equality of chest expansion
- Listen for cough (moist, dry, productive, or nonproductive)
- Check pulse oximetry
- Listen to apical pulse rate and rhythm
- Pay attention to blood pressure for hypotension or hypertension
- Evaluate blood pressure in both arms if indicated
- Evaluate wounds if present
- Check orthostatic vital signs if indicated (sitting and standing blood pressure and pulse)

---

be asked outright about the use of street drugs such as cocaine, methamphetamine, and heroin. Causes of chest pain in cocaine users include myocardial ischemia and infarction, myocarditis, aortic dissection, and pneumomediastinum. Because of the critical association between cocaine use and lethal cardiac complication from use, these patients should be considered for emergent care (Om et al., 1992). Because of the array of potential causes of chest pain, a more detailed physical assessment of the patient with chest pain may be necessary in triage, particularly in EDs with high-volume patient loads (Box 7–4). Besides obtaining vital signs, it is helpful to ascertain the patient's pulse oximetry for determination of a screening oxygenation status (Fig. 7–2). If a patient has a cool periphery, wears nail polish, or is breathing with a shallow depth, the accuracy of the oximetry reading may be affected. If possible, variables decreasing the accuracy should be eliminated. Ask the patient to slow the breathing and breath deeply, and reevaluate the oximetry reading if an initially low oxygen saturation value is seen. Professionals should also remember that oxygen saturation, as evaluated by pulse oximetry, may be excellent even when perfusion is grossly abnormal. To evaluate the patient fully, all screening assessment methods should be used in conjunction

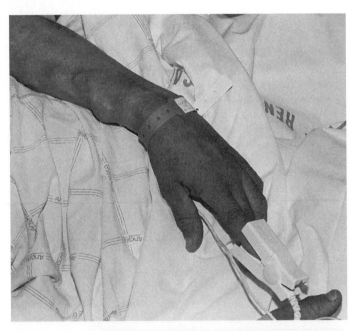

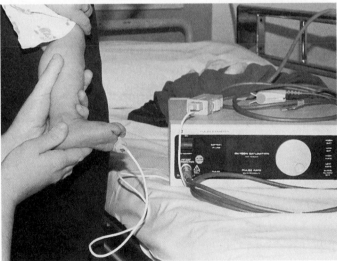

Fig. 7–2 **A,** Oxygenation may be assessed by obtaining O$_2$ saturation using a pulse oximeter. **B,** Pulse oximetry can be performed on a pediatric patient.

with the patient's history, general appearance, and other objective data.

Auscultation of the apical heart rate is helpful, especially in triage settings in which automatic blood pressure units are used to obtain blood pressure and pulse rates. Patients who have tachycardia or dysrhythmias that do not allow for forceful enough systolic contractions of the heart to cause a pulse pressure that is palpable in a peripheral pulse may wrongly be judged to have a lower pulse rate than is true. Ascertaining an apical pulse rate is useful not only in determining the patient's true pulse rate but also in giving the triage professional a quick understanding of the patient's hemodynamic stability based on the pulse deficit between apical and peripheral pulses (any difference greater than 4 is especially significant) (Fig. 7–3). Regularity of the apical rhythm should also be noted, with irregularities further assessed as being regularly irregular or ir-

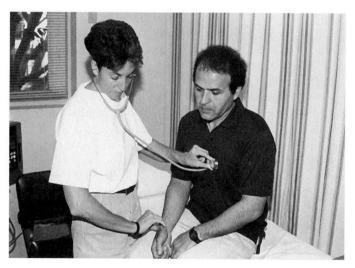

Fig. 7–3   Checking for a pulse deficit. Listening to the apical pulse while feeling the radial pulse will cue the nurse about the adequacy of systolic contractions in initiating a pressure wave sufficient to stimulate peripheral blood flow. The apical and radial pulses should be simultaneous (0.2 second difference in reality).

regularly irregular. Knowing whether there is a history of dysrhythmias, for example, atrial fibrillation, is helpful.

Observe the patient's skin for diaphoresis, pallor, cyanosis, or ashen color. If the patient is dark-skinned, look in the mouth at the oral mucosa for cyanosis and pallor. Ask significant others who have accompanied the patient whether they have observed a change in the patient's color. If respiratory compromise is a concern, listen to the patient's lungs. For patients who need immediate triage into the ED for care, the data that are normally collected in triage are obtained in the ED. The triage professional's skills and time should always be used for obtaining as valuable a data base on the patient as possible. When the patient is asked during the symptom analysis to indicate the location of chest pain, the triage professional should pay careful attention to how the patient identifies the location of the chest pain. If the patient can point to the area with one finger, it is often not a critical problem that is precipitating the pain. If the patient uses a fist and indicates the substernal area, this is called a positive Levine's sign and is associated with angina or myocardial infarction pain (Fig. 7–4). Because of the value of thrombolytic therapy and the potential for sudden death, the condition must be categorized as emergent and the patient triaged into the ED as rapidly as possible. In patients who have chest pain associated with dyspnea, the trachea should be assessed for midline position (one finger on the suprasternal notch), and the chest should be auscultated for bilateral breath sounds with a concern regarding the possibility of pneumothorax. This problem most often occurs in young, otherwise healthy men who have congenital pulmonary blebs, but it can also occur in persons with chronic asthma or those with an acute or past chest trauma or in those with lung cancer or other diseases affecting the lungs or pleural cavity. If the patient has a cough, it should be indicated whether the cough is productive or nonproductive; if the cough is productive, the characteristics of the sputum (hemoptysis, green, yellow, or clear) should be recorded.

If a patient arriving at triage is a diabetic (which is discovered because the patient indicates this immediately or it is revealed during the section of the triage interview related to medications or prior health problems), the triage professional remembers that many diabetics have neuropathy that may result in uncharacteristic or vague discomfort or pain, even in the pres-

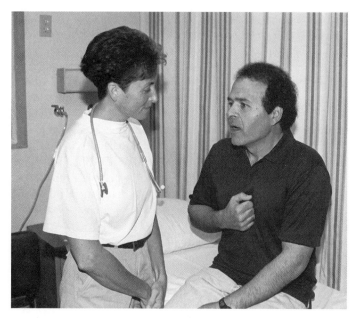

Fig. 7–4   Levine's sign is associated with angina or myocardial chest pain.

ence of acute coronary disease, and the patient should be triaged, according to this understanding, as "emergent." Diabetics, particularly those who are insulin dependent, are more than two times as likely as nondiabetic patients to have "silent ischemia" or cardiac events without chest pain (Naka et al., 1992). This may be a result of diabetics having lower levels of circulating beta-endorphins or neuropathy that affects the autonomic pain fibers innervating the heart (Hikita et al., 1993). Some diabetic patients seek emergency care not as a result of chest discomfort or cardiac complaints but as a result of complications of cardiac ischemia such as pulmonary edema (Roper et al., 1984).

In considering the many possible reasons for chest pain, triage professionals should keep in mind the association of various diagnoses with their most common precipitating factors (see Box 7–2) and pay close attention to interview response cues such as recent viral illness (pericarditis), cardiac surgery (Dressler's syndrome), fainting during or after exercise (idiopathic subaortic stenosis), history of acquired immunodeficiency disease (AIDS), pneumocystic pneumonia or cryptococcal pneumonia, or a family history of or recent exposure to contagious illnesses (tuberculosis). If dyspnea is an associated symptom, incorporating physical assessment techniques used for patients with dyspnea may also be necessary. Measurement of blood pressure in both arms may be indicated if an aneurysm is suspected. When triage or field personnel suspect the possibility of tuberculosis, it is imperative that they protect themselves by wearing tubercular-resistant face masks or placing a tubercular-resistant face mask over the patient, or both, to protect all people in the surrounding environment from the patient's respiratory droplets. In regions where specific health risks are increased, as with San Joaquin Valley fever, nurses must also stay informed of the signs and symptoms of prevalent diseases so that their knowledge base will be helpful in assessing and triaging patients accurately.

When evaluating the possibility that chest pain may be related to cardiac disease, the triage nurse may have to rely on more than just the patient's history and physical assessment data. It is important to understand the prevalence of coronary artery disease in various patient populations (Richards, 1992). To help determine whether the chest pain may be cardiac-related, patients may be asked about major risk factors. A high index of suspicion for pulmonary embolism should be present when individuals have risk factors for embolism such as recent orthopedic injuries or surgery or recent childbirth (Box 7–5).

Patients with chest pain who have had a rib fracture, whether from trauma or excessive coughing, or malignant pathology usually have pain that is localized to the affected area and is made worse with inspiration and coughing. They may also complain of a grating sensation during breathing and have localized tenderness on palpation of the affected area (Baum and Wolinsky, 1994).

Patients with tenderness in the chest wall associated with chest pain that is not related to cardiac disease usually have tenderness on palpation of the sternum, xiphoid process, left costosternal junctions, and left anterior chest wall (Wise et al., 1992). Palpation of these areas and general chest palpation

BOX 7–5	**Major Risk Factors for Pulmonary Embolism**

- Orthopedic surgery
- Long bone fracture
- Surgery
- Obesity
- Childbirth
- Aging
- Sedentary life-style
- Use of birth control pills

during triage may be accomplished most easily in male patients and if the triage area is discrete and may be helpful in determining the appropriate triage level for the patient with chest pain.

A high index of suspicion for pneumonia is cued when patients have dyspnea, chest pain, fever, and a cough. The acuity of the condition as evident in the patient's general appearance, pulse oximetry, degree of fever, and vital sign stability assists determination of the triage category. Other chest conditions with pulmonary and cardiac causes may be associated with fever, and the triage nurse should not assume that the patient with chest pain who has a fever has pneumonia. Fever, malaise, and chest pain are all common symptoms in patients with postmyocardial infarction syndrome, or Dressler's syndrome, and the triage nurse must realize that this syndrome may occur as late as several months after a myocardial infarction (Gregoratos, 1990). Dressler's syndrome may be more common in patients who have had an anterior myocardial infarction, but unless the patient arrives at triage with medical records this is only of theoretic interest (Sahasranam et al., 1990).

When there is a high index of suspicion for critical causes, patients who cannot receive treatment immediately should be kept in the triage area in as quiet an area as possible and in full view of the triage nurse. Periodic reassessment of these patients is mandatory.

Chest pain associated with chest trauma requires an emer-

BOX 7–6	Evaluation of Patients With Chest Trauma

- Mechanism of injury
- Type of trauma: For *penetrating trauma,* the direction and length of the instrument; for *gunshot,* the type of gun and bullet, and distance of patient from gun; for *blunt trauma,* the force, direction, and number of blows
- Time of injury
- Loss of consciousness
- Associated injuries
- Last food and fluid ingestion

---

gent evaluation and triage, often into the trauma care system (Box 7–6). The type of trauma (blunt or sharp) and time at which the trauma occurred should be ascertained immediately. Concurrently an evaluation of the patient's airway, respirations, and chest expansion for symmetry, adequacy, and depth and pulse oximetry should be performed, and vital signs should be obtained (Fig. 7–5). Penetrating wounds on the chest should be sealed with an occlusive dressing if tension pneumothorax is possible. As with patients who have emergent cardiac problems, the physical assessment of the chest trauma patient is best performed in the ED's trauma care center; however, if the patient is evaluated in a community setting or if entry into the ED is delayed, the triage professional makes use of the time by performing as thorough an evaluation as possible for the benefit of the patient. A history of blunt trauma to the chest, for example, impact from a baseball bat during an altercation, should be triaged and treated as a myocardial infarction, although pericardial effusion may be more likely, depending on the patient and degree of trauma. Patients with a history of penetrating trauma who arrive at triage with a knife or another instrument still in the chest should be triaged directly into the ED as emergent, but the sharp object should not be removed; it will be removed under surgeon's care. When a patient has been shot, it is helpful to learn (when appropriate and possible) what type of gun and bullet was used and how far from the gun the patient was when shot. The types of internal injuries are determined largely by

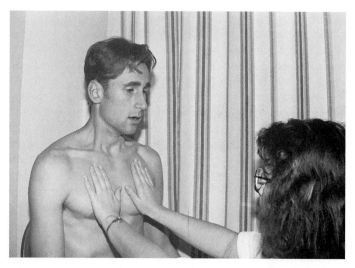

Fig. 7–5   If the patient's chest is exposed, the examiner can easily palpate the chest to assess for bilateral expansion.

bullet velocity, force, and distance. Because the triage professional may have more immediate contact with family or witnesses to the event, these persons should be interviewed for a careful history of the event and general information regarding the patient's allergies, prior health problems, last menstrual period (if a woman), and so forth. The triage professional then communicates this information to the trauma care staff. This is particularly urgent if the patient is unconscious. It is also helpful to determine the patient's last food and fluid ingestion if possible, since the patient may require surgery.

Patients with chest pain who have been exposed to smoke (smoke inhalation) or toxic chemical fumes should be triaged as emergent, since the condition has a high risk for deterioration without immediate oxygen therapy. Determination of the oxygen saturation, vital signs, and respiratory pattern is helpful, but these may need to be assessed by the ED staff. Information regarding the exposure should include the distance of the patient from the source of noxious fumes, known and greatest possible length of exposure, route of exposure (such as saturation of clothes), ventilation of the environment of exposure, and if possible, specific chemicals involved. Poison control and other resource agencies should be consulted as quickly as possible to obtain treatment advice for specific chemicals.

Patients with chest pain that is referred from the epigastrium and who have a history of ulcer or gastrointestinal bleeding should be asked questions about the presence and nature of their emesis and stools. Orthostatic vital signs should also be obtained (see Ulcers in Chapter 8). Gastrointestinal problems of esophageal motor abnormalities and reflux are found in the majority of patients who are admitted to the ED because of chest pain. Patients with chest pain should be asked whether they have a known history of these medical problems (Lam et al., 1992).

Patients who complain of chest pain and appear to be having a panic attack must be evaluated carefully, since the panic the patient exhibits may be the result of a true thoracic emergency and not a true panic disorder. Panic disorder affects 1% to 2% of the U.S. population and is frequently seen in ED patients (Beitman, 1992). Many patients with a history of panic disorder who have chest pain would in earlier times have had a diagnosis of neurocirculatory asthenia, which shares the symptoms of the new diagnosis: chest pain described as a dull ache near the cardiac apex, which may last from hours to days and is not related to effort, or as transient, stabbing chest pain near the cardiac apex. Patients may sigh frequently or complain that they feel that they are unable to breathe adequately. Accompanying symptoms include fatigue, palpitations, and

---

BOX 7–7	**Triage Treatment for Patients With Chest Pain**

- Rest
- Emesis basin
- Cool cloth for face if indicated
- Acetaminophen, if indicated, for oral temperature > 101° F
- Encouragement in relaxation and controlled breathing
- Education about triage process

---

multiple unexplained complaints in other body systems (Hurst, 1993). All patients with chest pain deserve careful evaluation with an understanding that patients who do not have critical vital signs or a chest pain pattern indicative of a true thoracic emergency may wait to be seen and will receive periodic reevaluations by the triage professional. Nonetheless, all patients with chest pain must have a brief but careful physical assessment before the triage designation is assigned (Box 7–7).

Palpitations

Some patients seeking emergency care may be free of chest pain but complain of palpitations. Unless ''quick-look'' monitoring is available in the triage area, it is difficult for the triage nurse to definitively diagnose the patient's cardiac rhythm. The triage nurse must make a determination of the seriousness of the patient's complaint based on a brief history, which specifically probes for accompanying symptoms such as syncope, diaphoresis, and chest pain; as well as the physical examination, which should include auscultation of the heart for an apical rate and rhythm and assessment of a pulse deficit (listening over the heart while palpating the radial pulse to determine whether every beat auscultated is felt at the radial pulse). A difference of more than four beats per minute may be significant, but careful evaluation of the apical pulse for rate and rhythm is even more crucial in determining whether the patient may have a life-threatening or serious dysrhythmia. One of the most critical associated symptoms to ask about is the presence of syncope. There are many cardiovascular causes of syncope (Box 7–8). Any patient who may have a life-threatening cardiac problem associated with syncope should be seen immediately in the ED for monitoring and therapeutic interventions. Idiopathic subaortic stenosis is a common cause of sudden death in athletes; it is important that the triage nurse be familiar with its hallmark signs, which may be seen in triage. These include dyspnea, syncope and dizziness, posteffort angina, jerky and brisk pulse, and a positive family history for sudden death (Marriott, 1993).

Patients with panic disorder are likely to describe their palpitations as ''racing'' or ''pounding'' and to be awakened from sleep by them, but these patients usually do not have life-threatening cardiac dysrhythmias; instead, they are more aware than

BOX 7–8	Cardiovascular and Hemodynamic Causes of Syncope*

- Complete heart block
- Ventricular tachycardia or fibrillation
- Idiopathic hypertrophic subaortic stenosis
- Mitral stenosis and atrial fibrillation
- Aortic stenosis
- Blood loss
- Myocardial infarction
- Pulmonary embolism
- Dissecting aneurysm
- Sick sinus syndrome

*Often accompanied by complaint of ''palpitations.''

most people of their body and are likely to have panic attacks that are precipitated by sensations such as tachycardia and dyspnea (Barsky et al., 1994).

RESPIRATORY PROBLEMS
Dyspnea

Dyspnea may be caused by pulmonary or cardiac diseases, or it may be associated with traumatic or other systemic disorders. During the interview and physical examination triage nurses should consider all possible causes of dyspnea and customize history questions to determine an appropriate triage level for the patient (Box 7–9).

Airway Obstruction and Choking

Patients who enter triage with difficulty in breathing may have a true threat to airway integrity or oxygenation. The triage professional's first assessment of a patient with dyspnea should be evaluation of the patency of the individual's airway. If the patient has stridorous respirations (crowing or high-pitched sounds during breathing), the professional will be alert to the potential for airway obstruction.

Inflammatory processes such as epiglottitis, laryngeal trauma, and laryngeal tumors, as well as systemic diseases such

| BOX 7–9 | Causes of Dyspnea |

ACUTE

Upper airway obstruction (laryngospasm, aspirated foreign body, neoplasm)

Asthma

Chest trauma (rib fracture, pneumothorax, lung contusion, vascular rupture, bronchial rupture)

Pneumonia (pleural effusion may contribute)

Pulmonary embolism

Acute interstitial lung disease (hemorrhage, adult respiratory distress syndrome)

Cardiogenic pulmonary edema

Spontaneous pneumothorax

CHRONIC

Chronic obstructive pulmonary disease

Cystic fibrosis

Interstitial lung diseases

Pleural effusion

Fibrothorax

Abnormalities of chest wall (kyphoscoliosis, neuromuscular disease, diaphragmatic paralysis)

Pulmonary vascular disease (primary pulmonary hypertension, organizing pulmonary emboli, venoocclusive disease, vascular malformations)

Cardiovascular disease

Severe anemia

Psychogenic dyspnea

From Baum G, Wolinsky E, eds: *Textbook of pulmonary diseases,* ed 5, Boston, 1994, Little, Brown.

as Wegener's granulomatosis and sarcoidosis, may be responsible for acute upper airway obstruction that is not related to choking caused by a bolus (Lerner and Deeb, 1993). If airway obstruction is observed, no matter what the cause, the patient needs immediate triage into an area where assessment for and removal of a foreign body (if present) can take place. Even in patients who have a less dramatic presentation of airway obstruction but who have airway compromise, assessment and optimization of the airway should be concurrent. General assessment of airway patency and integrity is accomplished by observing the thorax for bilateral chest expansion, placing a hand or finger under the patient's mouth or nose or both to feel for the movement of air, and auscultating the chest for exchange of air. As taught in basic cardiopulmonary resuscitation, an individual who appears to have difficulty breathing but who can cough effectively should not be disturbed. If the individual continues to choke and is not coughing effectively or is becoming pallid or cyanotic, assistance should be given to clear the airway immediately. Back blows, chest thrusts, and the Heimlich maneuver are all options for mechanically assisting clearance of an obstructed airway. The patient should be triaged into the ED as "emergent," since visualization of the item obstructing the patient's airway is possible and removal of foreign objects or a food bolus is facilitated by the use of Magill forceps. Many objects have been responsible for airway obstruction. It is helpful if the triage nurse can determine what the object might be, from individuals accompanying the patient. This information can be important, for instance, if the object is a drug package (e.g., cocaine), since rupture of the package may lead to overdose following or concurrent with airway difficulties (Ortega and Halterman, 1993).

If the patient comes to prehospital personnel in a field situation, efforts are made to clear the airway before transporting the patient, and clearance of the airway is achieved immediately, if possible. If the patient arrives at a school or clinic, emergency measures are initiated concurrently with calling for an ambulance. Patients who are choking victims should be transported to an acute care facility, even if the airway is cleared, for evaluation of the airway for trauma and possible assessment for aspiration pneumonia. Predisposing risk factors for bolus aspiration should be considered in triage and when teaching all patients who are at risk. These factors include severe psychiatric illness, abnormal eating behavior, local or spread-brain lesions, dysphagia, old age, multimorbidity, and newly institutionalized persons (Schmitt and Hewer, 1993). In elderly patients large fruit pits commonly lodge in the upper esophagus, compressing the trachea and thereby causing upper airway obstruction as a result of dysphagia, central nervous system disease, or alcohol ingestion (Dailey et al., 1992). Adult epiglottitis should also be considered, particularly in patients who have difficulty with swallowing their saliva and who have a fever and muffled voice. Other common causes of upper airway obstruction are listed in Box 7–10, which can be used as a guide for triage classification.

Choking may result from foreign bodies or food boluses occluding the airway, but it may also be the result of tumors, gross edema, or other medical conditions that require invasive evaluation and treatment. When it is clear that a foreign body is not causing the signs and symptoms of choking, the patient

---

| BOX 7–10 | Causes of Upper Airway Obstruction |

CHRONIC CONDITIONS
- Tumors
- Congenital malformations or dysfunctions
- Subglottic stenosis
- Chronic inflammatory diseases
- Sleep apnea syndrome
- Infections of oropharynx
- High-esophageal foreign bodies
- Stevens-Johnson syndrome
- Croup and tracheitis

ACUTE CONDITIONS LIKELY TO REQUIRE IMMEDIATE EVALUATION AND TREATMENT
- Burns (thermal or chemical)
- Hematomas resulting from warfarin therapy
- Epiglottitis
- Angioneurotic edema
- Laryngospasm
- Foreign body

Modified from Dailey R et al: *The airway: emergency management,* St Louis, 1992, Mosby.

should be transported and treated quickly and calmly, to prevent emotional outbursts by the patient, which may further challenge the airway. Cricothryoidotomy may be necessary. If a designated area in the ED exists for airway emergencies, the patient should be triaged directly to that area. Any person who is dyspneic because of choking deserves triage into an acute care area for airway management, since this emergency may cause death.

In pediatric patients gastroesophageal reflux is a common cause of stridor and may also cause recurrent croup, exacerbation of subglottic stenosis, laryngeal irritation with or without laryngospasm, chronic cough, and obstructive apnea. Parents of children with obstructive airway symptoms should be asked in triage whether the child has a history of gastroesophageal reflux (Burton et al., 1992). Any cause of airway obstruction is more critical in children than in adults because of the relatively small airway in children, which is more easily restricted or occluded by mucus, blood, or edema. Observation of children with airway obstruction or challenge will reveal tachypnea and retraction, which are best observed by removing the child's shirt to view the chest. The chest may have referred upper airway noise, which may include stridor. Children who are conscious should be allowed to assume a position of comfort; those with a diminished level of consciousness should assume the sniffing position or jaw-thrust position while being brought into the ED for care (Soud, 1992).

Asthmatic Crisis

Hospitalization rates for patients with asthma appear to be increasing worldwide (Weiss and Stein, 1992). Pediatric and adult patients with asthma have difficulty in breathing because of outflow obstruction of the airway—bronchi and bronchioles become inflamed and prevent the effective exhalation of air. When the asthma is appropriately managed, many individuals such as world-renowned athlete Jackie Joyner-Kersee live active, productive lives despite their asthma. Asthmatic crises may be rare in these individuals or may occur often during particularly difficult seasons, for example, during the summer when the weather is hot and in cities when pollution levels are high. Other patients, despite optimal management, are prone to asthmatic crises because of the nature and severity of their dis-

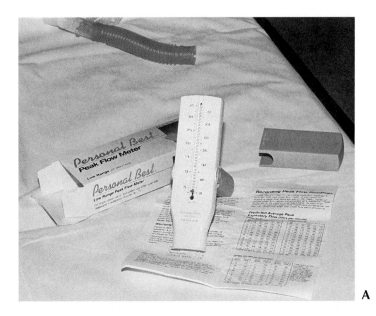

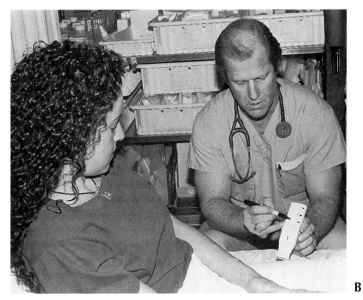

Fig. 7–6 **A,** Peak flow measurement device. **B,** It is important to explain the procedure for obtaining a peak flow measurement.

ease. Although emotional upsets may precipitate the symptoms of asthma, the effects of the disease are real. Patients who have dyspnea and oxygenation compromise as a result of asthma may die if acute, aggressive treatment is not available when needed.

Triage of the individual who is having an asthmatic crisis involves assessment of the degree of the dyspnea as it affects oxygenation and consideration of early treatment to effect bronchodilation and improvement in ventilation and perfusion. If the individual is able to speak in sentences, it is likely that there is sufficient time to complete the triage process and initiate respiratory measures to effect bronchodilation. In addition to evaluating the patient's ability to breathe and speak, the professional should assess the patient for use of accessory muscles, sternal retractions, cyanosis, and pallor. Pulse oximetry is useful in evaluating the patient's oxygen saturation levels, and results should be recorded. Measurement of the patient's peak end-expiratory flow volume may be useful in establishing the severity of the patient's crisis; such an assessment is helpful in providing a baseline understanding of the patient's respiratory

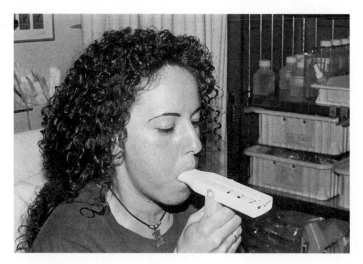

Fig. 7–7   The patient is encouraged to exhale in a forceful "blast" to obtain the true peak flow.

status (Figs. 7–6 and 7–7). If hemodynamic compromise is suspected, assessment of the apical pulse may be necessary to establish the patient's true pulse rate.

The physical assessment of the patient in asthmatic crises, with particular attention to the patient's airway and breathing norms is paramount, but a history of the patient's present illness should not be omitted. The history should be obtained, whenever possible, from family or friends accompanying the patient, to avoid tiring the patient and increasing the respiratory rate and dyspnea by requiring the patient to talk when she/he must breathe with great effort (Box 7–11). If the patient's crisis is related to an acute allergic reaction, this information should be provided to the medical staff immediately so that appropriate orders may be given.

If the patient is responding to an animal allergen, the patient's hands should be washed to remove animal dander, and clothing that has been exposed to the animal's hair should be removed. Patients who seek medical care from professionals outside hospital settings should receive immediate treatment (when available) for their particular problem (e.g., EpiPen or inhalers) (Fig. 7–8). Access to emergency transportation should not be delayed if the patient's asthmatic condition is escalating to the point where oxygenation is critically compromised (Box 7–12).

BOX 7–11	**Key Data To Obtain in Interview of Patients With Asthma**

- Determination of time and manner of onset of asthma
- Identification of incitants to the crisis, such as allergens, viral respiratory infection, air pollutants, exposure to toxins, cool air, temperature or humidity changes
- Medication use, including breathing treatments used at home and aerosolized medications and their effectiveness and last dosage time (Pay attention to underuse of medications and use of medications that may precipitate asthma.)
- Does the patient smoke cigarettes? Use other forms of tobacco, marijuana, or clove cigarettes?

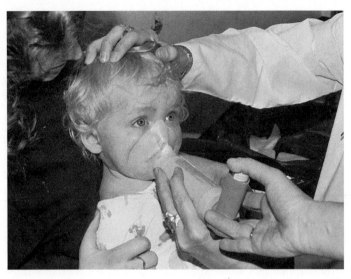

Fig. 7–8 Pediatric aerochamber devices maximize the delivery of inhalant medication.

BOX 7–12	**Clinical Signs and Symptoms of Asthmatic Crisis**

- Diminished level of consciousness
- Central cyanosis
- Severe respiratory distress or exhaustion
- Recurrent acute episodes over a short period, e.g., 2 to 7 days
- Increasing bronchodilatory requirement with minimal relief
- Profuse diaphoresis
- Wheezing on inspiration or silent chest
- Tachypnea, respiratory rate > 30 breaths/min
- Tachycardia, heart rate > 120 beats/min
- Peak expiratory flow rate < 100 to 200 l/min or < 25% to 50% of predicted value

Modified from Weiss E, Stein M, eds: *Bronchial asthma: mechanisms and therapeutics,* ed 3, Boston, 1993, Little, Brown.

| BOX 7–13 | **Risk Factors for Death in Patients With Asthma** |

DEMOGRAPHIC FACTORS

Adolescent or young adult
Non-Caucasian

HISTORICAL FACTORS

Prior life-threatening attacks (prior intubation for asthma)
Hospitalizations or emergency room visits (three or more) within
    past year
Use of three or more drugs for treatment of asthma
Airway lability (PEFR)
Corticosteroid use (past and present)
History of syncope or hypoxic seizures
Coexisting severe lung disease

PSYCHOSOCIAL FACTORS

Poor compliance with medications or inability to use treatment
    devices
Denial
Alcoholism
Continued smoking
Depression or other major psychiatric illness
Procrastination in seeking medical care

PHYSICIAN-RELATED FACTORS

Failure to diagnose or appreciate severity of attack
Underuse of corticosteroids
Failure to adequately follow up and monitor the case by means of
    objective measures
Inappropriate use of sedatives or other drugs
Failure to identify high-risk patient
Failure to educate patient

From Weiss E, Stein M, eds: *Bronchial asthma: mechanisms and therapeutics,*
ed 3, Boston, 1993, Little, Brown.

If during the history the triage nurse discovers the presence of psychiatric diagnoses or noncompliance with therapeutic regimen for asthma, or both, the nurse should be aware that the patient's risk for potentially fatal asthma is greater, since these two factors have been identified as common features in patients who die during an asthmatic crisis (Miller et al., 1992). Other risk factors for death in patients with asthma are presented in Box 7–13.

Because it is frightening to not feel able to breathe, it is important that patients in asthmatic crisis be handled calmly and deftly. Hypoxia causes agitation and emotional lability in many patients, and when hypoxia is suspected or determined to be present, oxygen therapy should be initiated aggressively as early as possible. For the patient with chronic asthma who has chronic pulmonary disease, special consideration may be necessary when delivering oxygen therapy and following medical

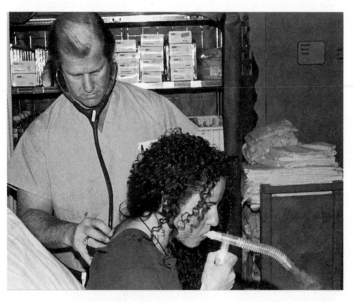

Fig. 7–9   Respiratory treatments may be given immediately after triage or in field care to alleviate acute outflow obstruction in patients with acute asthma or bronchitis. Assessment is often concurrent with therapy.

orders regarding the amount of oxygen delivered (Fig. 7–9). Asthmatics who arrive at triage who have not used their inhalers correctly or recently should be encouraged to do so if the facility's triage protocols recommend this. It is helpful to use a spacer in conjunction with inhalers for effective medication delivery.

Inhalation of Toxins

Patients who have inhaled toxins may or may not arrive at triage with a clear history of having done so. If it is clear that the event precipitating the emergent or presenting condition involved inhaling toxins (e.g., smoke inhalation), it is easier to perform a system-specific examination and identify the appropriate triage category. If, however, the patient is not sure of the cause of the symptoms, a careful eye to the possibility that the patient has inhaled toxins is necessary when indicated by the history, signs, or symptoms of the patient.

During the triage history the possibility that the patient has inhaled toxins should be considered if the patient reports a vague feeling of malaise progressing over a period of hours or days and discussion of the patient's home environment yields information consistent with toxic fumes. Toxins patients are sometimes unknowingly exposed to include carbon monoxide, which is especially troublesome because the ultimate consequence may be severe hypoxia and death and it is impossible to identify in the environment by smell, since it is a colorless and odorless gas. Attention should be paid when individuals working in occupations where they are exposed to chemicals report suspected symptoms of toxic fume inhalation. These occupations include homemaking, since homemakers may be exposed to potentially dangerous combinations of cleaning fluids such as bleach and ammonia or they may be exposed to paint fumes when redecorating or painting. Another common problem in EDs is patient exposure to pest fumigation. Patients who reenter a home or business before the prescribed time for entering a fumigated area expose themselves to a dangerous level of fumes. Some patients report that they stayed home but closed off areas that were fumigated. When patients have been exposed to fumes, it is helpful to determine the duration of exposure, the chemical they have inhaled, and the area and ventilation of the environment. Underventilation or lack of

ventilation increases the patient's risk of consequences of toxic
fume inhalation, and the history should include questions about
the ventilation of the patient's environment during exposure to
the toxic fume. Patients who work in paid occupations with
chemical fume exposure should be asked about the use of respirators during contact with toxic fumes, and they should be
asked to describe the equipment used. There are many types of
respirators, and some patients may consider a simple mask to
be a respirator or protective against fumes, which is not true.
Farming is another occupation with extremely high risk for inhalation injuries resulting from work in grain silos and manure
pits and from barn and tobacco dust.

Smoke inhalation may be seen separately from or in conjunction with facial or thoracic burns. Patients who do not report
a history of smoke inhalation because they are agitated, anxious,
confused, or have an altered level of consciousness should be
examined for signs and symptoms of smoke inhalation. These
include singed nasal hairs, black-tinged sputum, adventitious
lung sounds, cough, hoarseness, and hypoxia. The triage nurse
should delay triage of the patient with a history of smoke inhalation only long enough to obtain vital signs and essential
historical data related to allergies and medications. Remaining
questions usually asked during full triage should be deferred for
the ED personnel caring for the patient, since a complete oxygenation assessment and oxygen therapy are immediately necessary for the best possible patient outcome.

Restrictive Pulmonary Disease

The patient who has chronic pulmonary problems such as
pleural effusion is usually quick to inform the triage professional, to access the most appropriate care as soon as possible.
Patients with a history of pulmonary fibrosis or tuberculosis
who have restrictive pulmonary disease are also often astute at
giving the triage nurse their history so that appropriate measures
may be taken to evaluate the acuity of their presenting status
for appropriate triage. Many patients, however, do not provide
information immediately that is helpful in understanding that
the patient suffers from restrictive pulmonary disease; these patients benefit from a professional who is quick to recognize the
signs and symptoms of restrictive pulmonary problems and who

will communicate the patient's concerns to care-providing professionals to whom the patient will be triaged.

Pulmonary Edema

Triage professionals and those familiar with emergency and cardiac care are familiar with the typical pattern in cardiac patients prone to pulmonary edema. The clock on night shift rolls to 2 A.M. and when an emergency call is received, one of the likely reasons is to summon care for an individual who has awakened with severe dyspnea, cough, and hypoxia. Care of individuals with pulmonary edema is based on rapid recognition of its hallmark signs and symptoms: dyspnea, tachypnea, accessory muscle use, neck vein distention (particularly when pulmonary edema coexists with right-sided heart failure), tachycardia, moist rales, a dry cough, and a feeling of panic. All patients who arrive at triage with this problem require immediate care and should not be delayed in triage. If field care is initiated, treatment should be efficiently directed at relieving the patient of circulatory overload and perfusion compromise by rapid delivery of oxygen, morphine, and diuretics and by maintaining the patient in Fowler's position. If a patient arrives at triage with pulmonary edema that is not fulminant, assessment measures to determine the patient's oxygenation status and level of perfusion should be performed.

RESPIRATORY PATTERN PROBLEMS
Respiratory Depression

One of the first assessments to be performed in triage is vital sign measurement (Box 7–14). If during the course of assessing

BOX 7–14	**Triage Treatment of Patients With Respiratory Ailments**

- Provide as quiet an environment as possible
- Encourage relaxation and concentration on efficient respirations
- Provide portable oxygen if indicated and available
- Encourage appropriate use of inhalers if indicated
- Maintain patient in position of comfort (upright)

a patient's vital signs it is observed that the patient is brady-pneic, respiratory depression should be suspected. The patient's respiratory pattern should also be closely observed to determine whether the examiner has assessed the patient's respiratory rate correctly and to begin to get a more complete picture of the patient's respiratory status. Respiratory rate in patients who are thoracic breathers may be easier to evaluate than in patients who are abdominal or en bloc (combination thoracic and abdominal) breathers. To determine how to observe or where to inconspic-uously rest your pulse-taking hand, ask the patient to take a deep breath while assessing the patient's respiratory rate. The rhythm, depth, and inspiration/expiration ratio of the patient's breathing should also be observed, as for all respiratory prob-lems. When respiratory depression is suspected, the triage pro-fessional should follow the usual measures in assessing the patient's oxygenation status (Box 7–15). One of the most common causes of respiratory depression is narcotic ingestion, overdose, or intolerance. Obtaining a careful medication history is important, with a careful eye toward narcotic medications, the amount or dosage ingested, the patient's last dose, total recent doses, and tolerance based on critical medical problems such as renal failure. If a patient denies narcotic ingestion, the patient's response is recorded.

Nurses and other health care professionals should be astute in observing signs of street drug use such as the presence of needle track marks. It should be routine to ask patients about

BOX 7–15	**Evaluation of Patient Oxygenation Status**

- Assess vital signs (watch for tachypnea, tachycardia)
- Observe for pallor, cyanosis, ashen skin, skin changes
- Observe for signs of increased respiratory effort (use of accessory muscles, sternal retractions)
- Perform pulse oximetry (<90% is critical)
- Listen for stridor
- Auscultate chest for diminished or absent breath sounds
- Auscultate chest for adventitious breath sounds (wheezing, rhonchi, crackles)

the use of street or recreational drugs. It is not unusual for ED personnel to care for individuals who have taken an overdose of heroin. Again, experience makes the recognition of this problem probable in a short time; signs include pinpoint pupils, respiratory depression or arrest, track marks, or other obvious signs of intravenous drug use. Of course, any patient with respiratory depression resulting in respiratory arrest or unconsciousness must be triaged immediately for care, but the triage professional can be helpful by obtaining information about the individual's medications and allergies from significant others.

Aside from narcotics or chronic respiratory problems in acute exacerbation, another cause of respiratory depression is the presence of a brain tumor. A watchful eye in triage for the patient's neurologic stability is helpful, and a mini-neurologic assessment should be incorporated if anything seems amiss and relevant to the respiratory depression observed in the patient. Assessments of the patient's gait, pupils, symmetry of movements, speech, and level of consciousness are relatively easy to quickly incorporate into the observations performed in triage. If the patient is alert, care should still be taken to assess the patient's orientation to time, place, and person. Again, any concern relevant to the patient's oxygenation status warrants a rapid assessment of oxygenation. A Glasgow Coma Scale score should be obtained for patients with drug overdoses and brain tumors. Other causes of respiratory depression include hypothermia and diabetic ketoacidosis. These causes are most easily discovered during the history and confirmed by obtaining vital signs or by a rapid glucose level test. Patients with these conditions should be triaged immediately for care, since corrective measures are definitive and cannot be initiated easily in the triage area. If the patient with diabetic ketoacidosis must wait and is not vomiting, she/he should be encouraged to drink water to help dilute the glucose in the bloodstream and begin the glucose reduction process.

Patients in triage who have respiratory depression should be encouraged to breathe deeply and consistently while awaiting treatment. In maximizing the patient's respiratory performance, coaching from family members can also be elicited when helpful.

Pneumothorax

Pneumothorax may occur in patients with spontaneous lung deflation and in patients who have had a traumatic injury or illness affecting the pleural space or lungs, such as cancer. Recognizing the hallmarks of pneumothorax is helpful because prompt treatment can be initiated, thereby preventing complications from pneumothorax such as a mediastinal shift and death. If the triage nurse intuitively suspects pneumothorax soon after seeing the patient, it may be helpful to ask whether the patient has ever had similar symptoms and had the diagnosis of a lung abnormality before. In almost all patients with primary spontaneous pneumothorax (PSP) the rate of recurrence is 30% to 50% within 5 years. The most common cause of pneumothorax is a spontaneous congenital bleb rupture, usually in young men who are smokers. Family history of PSP is also significant in many individuals. Pneumothorax is increasingly seen in patients with AIDS, particularly in large urban areas, and is associated with a high mortality rate. In AIDS patients with PSP the most common associated infection is *Pneumocystis carinii* pneu-

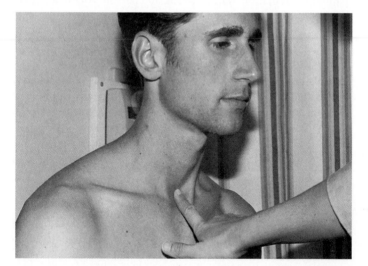

Fig. 7–10   Feeling for the patient's trachea as midline in the suprasternal notch is a rapid method for detecting tracheal deviation.

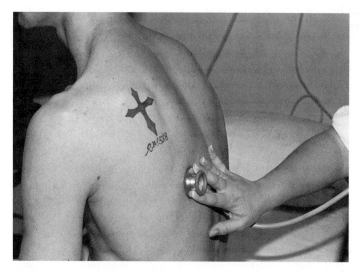

Fig. 7–11   Auscultation of the posterior thorax allows the most extensive surface assessment of the lung periphery.

monia. Complaints of patients with pneumothorax include sudden or increasingly severe chest pain, dyspnea, and agitation. Using one finger to palpate the trachea at the suprasternal notch, the triage professional can rapidly assess for tracheal deviation (Fig. 7–10). Assessment of the chest for bilateral expansion with respirations is also useful, and auscultating the chest for bilateral breath sounds anteriorly and posteriorly over the major thoracic auscultatory areas is imperative during evaluation for pneumothorax (Fig. 7–11). Patients with a history of pneumothorax automatically have a higher risk for pneumothorax. When an obvious case of pneumothorax exists, the patient should not be delayed in triage or, if this is discovered outside an acute care facility, in the field. Chest tube insertion for lung reinflation without delay is usually required.

TRAUMA
Gunshot Wounds

Patients with trauma to the thorax as a result of a gunshot wound are immediately triaged into the ED or trauma care area for a full evaluation. Since ensuring this course of action may be the responsibility of the triage professional, particularly when patients are driven to the ED by private vehicle, it is important, once the patient has been triaged into the ED, for the triage nurse to obtain as much vital information as possible if this is within her/his role expectations. Critical general information that should be communicated to trauma care professionals as quickly as possible includes information about the patient's allergies to medications, medical problems, and daily medications. If possible, it is also helpful to find out what type of weapon was used, the distance of the patient from the weapon, the type of ammunition, and whether the event precipitating the patient's injury was homicidal or suicidal. Designated personnel will contact the appropriate law enforcement agency. When the patient has participated in a violent altercation, security measures should be in place in the ED to protect ED personnel from reprisals or gang warfare. Furthermore, it is important to save and search all clothing for the presence of weapons so that they can be handled and stored safely. When it is discovered that a patient has suffered a gunshot wound as a result of an intended act of suicide, all personnel should do their utmost to ensure that the patient is admitted, since the lethal nature of that mode of action indicates that the patient is a serious risk to himself/herself.

Stab Wounds or Penetrating Trauma

Patients who receive stab wounds or penetrating trauma may have superficial or critical injuries. A rapid assessment of patients with this history is necessary. Because of hemodynamic compensation, the patient sometimes arrives at triage with perfect vital signs, yet these deteriorate rapidly if internal injuries that result in persistent internal hemorrhaging are present. An evaluation of the patient's wound(s) must be made while the triage professional is obtaining the patient's vital signs. For a knife wound it is helpful to know the type and size of the knife and the mode of injury. If the patient has been violently stabbed it is useful to know whether the perpetrator is male or female. Women who stab tend to insert the knife down into the patient's upper thorax, whereas men often stab upward into the patient's diaphragm and abdomen. Men tend to inflict more lethal wounds, although either type of stab wounds can cause critical injuries when the length of the knife and force of the stabbing are sufficient to enter critical organs, major blood vessels, or other anatomic structures. Again, for the protection of emergency personnel, it is useful to determine immediately whether there should be a security alert. This precaution is most common when the perpetrator who inflicted the injuries is not in custody or when gang involvement is suspected or known. Once the patient's wounds have been checked, the nurse should apply a sterile dressing over the wounds. If a sucking chest wound is evident, an occlusive dressing should be applied immediately to prevent a tension pneumothorax (Fig. 7–12). Immediate assessment of the patient's pulmonary integrity should be deferred to the ED personnel, although auscultation of the chest for breath sounds may be helpful in determining the likelihood that chest tubes or intubation should be prepared for use.

When the patient has received an accidental stab wound, such as from a flying sharp object in a car during an accident

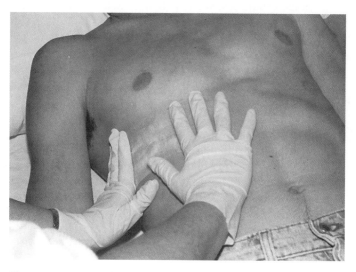

Fig. 7–12   An occlusive dressing is applied over any puncture wound (penetrating trauma) with the potential for creating a tension pneumothorax.

or from accidental stabbing during cooking with a kitchen knife or accidental stabbing from an X-ACTO knife (used for art) or other occupational implement, there is less likelihood of critical injuries, since the force of the stabbing and the length of the implement are usually less than in a violent stabbing. Triage of these patients should be brief but thorough. Because of the mechanism of the injury, emergent triage status will be assigned, even when the patient's condition is stable at the time of triage.

Fractured Ribs or Sternum

Fractures involving the skeletal structures of the thorax may cause pneumothorax, flail chest, myocardial injuries, pericardial tamponade, or simply severe chest pain. Mechanisms of injury that cause fractures include blunt trauma such as the patient's chest hitting the steering wheel, baseball bat to the chest (intentional or accidental), kicking of the chest (sports related or violence related), or pathologic fractures involving, for example, osteoporosis or cancer lesions. In any case, no matter what the cause is, because of the aforementioned consequences the triage professional should assess any patient at risk for skeletal fractures for the presence of such fractures. Triage status is designated according to the complications already evident or the potential for problems resulting from the severity of the patient's pain, compromise in oxygenation, or age. Flail chest (paradoxic chest wall motion during breathing that results from sequential, double fractures of three or more ribs, which causes a free-floating segment of chest wall) occurs in 1 of 13 patients with rib fractures and has a mortality rate of 5% to 50% (Dailey et al., 1992). Auscultation of the chest for bilateral breath sounds may reveal crepitation or popping during respirations as fractured segments of a rib rub against each other. Tenderness to palpation may also raise the professional's index of suspicion that the patient has a fractured rib or sternum. Flail chest also causes paradoxic movement of the flail segment, increased splinting, and decreased cough effectiveness (Dailey et al., 1992).

Assessment of the patient's pulse in the event of all thoracic injuries should include auscultation of the patient's apical pulse, since a pulse deficit may exist and cardiac auscultation may be the first opportunity to suspect pericardial tamponade if the heart sounds are discovered to be very different. The nurse who suspects pericardial tamponade should assess the patient for Beck's triad: distended neck veins, narrow pulse pressure, and distant heart sounds. Pericardial tamponade occurs in patients with penetrating trauma or severe blunt trauma to the chest and after cardiac surgery or myocardial infarction in patients who have Dressler's syndrome, an inflammatory rather than traumatic-induced tamponade. All patients with respiratory or hemodynamic compromise are triaged as emergent. Those who must wait for treatment receive, at least, periodic reassessment of vital signs and pulse oximetry. They should be kept in full view of the triage professional, who continues to monitor the patient's skin for color, diaphoresis, and other changes that indicate a deterioration in the patient's condition.

Pulmonary Contusion

Patients with trauma to the chest may have damage to lung tissue, or pulmonary contusion. Since this problem may not be immediately evident, the ''walk-in'' trauma patient entering triage who has had a significant injury to the chest should be considered at risk for pulmonary contusion. If evidence exists that this may be a risk, the patient should be triaged for emergent care since, despite advances in pulmonary care, patients with pulmonary contusion and flail chest continue to have a morbidity and mortality rate of 13% to 50%. Clinical signs and symptoms may include evidence of chest wall trauma (ecchymoses or erythema), pain, dyspnea, tachypnea, hypotension, and in half of all patients with this problem, hemoptysis (Dailey et al., 1992).

REFERENCES

Barsky A et al: Panic disorder, palpitations, and the awareness of cardiac activity, *J Nerv Ment Dis* 182(2):63, 1994.

Baum G, Wolinsky E, eds: *Textbook of pulmonary diseases,* ed 5, Boston, 1994, Little, Brown.

Beitman B: Panic disorder in patients with angiographically normal coronary arteries, *Am J Med* 92(5A):335, 1992.

Burton D et al: Pediatric airway manifestations of gastroesophageal reflux, *Ann Otol Rhinol Laryngol* 101(9):742, 1992.

Dailey R et al: *The airway: emergency management,* St Louis, 1992, Mosby.

Gregoratos G: Pericardial involvement in acute myocardial infarction, *Cardiol Clin* 8(4):601, 1990.

Hikita H et al: Usefulness of plasma beta-endorphin level, pain threshold and autonomic function in assessing silent myocardial ischemia in patients with and without diabetes mellitus, *Am J Cardiol* 72(2):140, 1993.

Hurst W: *Cardiovascular diagnosis:the initial examination,* St Louis, 1993, Mosby.

Lam H et al: Acute noncardiac chest pain in a coronary care unit: evaluation by 24-hour pressure and pH recording of the esophagus, *Gastroenterology* 102(2):453, 1992.

Lerner D, Deeb Z: Acute upper airway obstruction resulting from systemic diseases, *South Med J* 86(6):623, 1993.

Marriott H: *Bedside cardiac diagnosis,* Philadelphia, 1993, Lippincott.

Miller T, Greenberger P, Patterson R: The diagnosis of potentially fatal asthma in hospitalized adults: patient characteristics and increased severity of asthma, *Chest* 102(2):515, 1992.

Naka M et al: Silent myocardial ischemia in patients with non-insulin-dependent diabetes mellitus as judged by treadmill exercise testing and coronary angiography, *Am Heart J* 123(1):46, 1992.

Om A et al: Frequency of coronary artery disease and left ventricle dysfunction in cocaine users, *Am J Cardiol* 69(29):1549, 1992.

Ortega R, Halterman M: Concealed illegal drugs: a potential cause of airway obstruction, *Anesth Analg* 76(1):204, 1993.

Richards S: Atypical chest pain: differentiation from coronary artery disease, *Postgrad Med* 91(5):257, 263, 1992.

Roper et al: The syndrome of sudden severe painless myocardial ischemia, *Am Heart J* 107:813, 1984.

Sahasranam K, Chandra P, Ravindran K: Early onset Dressler's syndrome: a study of fifteen cases, *Indian J Chest Dis Allied Sci* 32(3):153, 1990.

Schmitt M, Hewer W: Life-threatening situations caused by bolus aspiration in psychiatric inpatients: clinical aspects, risk factors, prevention, therapy, *Fortschr Neurol Psychiatr* 61(9):313, 1993.

Soud T: Airway, breathing, circulation, and disability: what is different about kids? *J Emerg Nurs* 18(2):107, 1992.

Weiss E, Stein M, eds: *Bronchial asthma: mechanisms and therapeutics,* ed 3, Boston, 1993, Little, Brown.

Wise C, Semble E, Dalton C: Musculoskeletal chest wall syndromes in patients with noncardiac chest pain: a study of 100 patients, *Arch Med Rehabil* 73(2):147, 1992.

RECOMMENDED READING

Baum G, Wolinsky E, eds: *Textbook of pulmonary diseases,* ed 5, Boston, 1994, Little, Brown.

Boltz MA: Nurse's guide to identifying cardiac rhythms, *Nursing* 24(4):54, 1994.

Braunwald E, ed: *Heart disease: a textbook of cardiovascular medicine,* ed 4, Philadelphia, 1992, WB Saunders.

Cohn P: *Silent myocardial ischemia and infarction,* ed 3, New York, 1993, Marcel Dekker.

Finesilver C: Respiratory assessment, *RN* Feb, 1992.

Goldberger E: *Treatment of cardiac emergencies,* ed 5, St Louis, 1990, Mosby.

Green E: Solving the puzzle of chest pain, *Am J Nurs* 92(1):32, 1992.

Hurst W: *Cardiovascular diagnosis: the initial examination,* St Louis, 1993, Mosby.

Kaplan N: *Clinical hypertension,* ed 6, Baltimore, 1994, Williams & Wilkins.

Miller A, Harvey J: Guidelines for the management of spontaneous pneumothorax. Standards of Care Committee of the British Thoracic Society, *Br Med J* 307(6899):308, 1993 (published erratum).

Povenmire K, House M: Recognizing the cocaine addict, *Nursing 90* 20:46, 1990.

8 | Abdominal, Rectal, and Genital Problems

Patient complaints dealing with the abdomen can have single, multiple, and diverse ramifications. Housed within this anatomic area are organs responsible for digestion, elimination, reproduction, immunologic function, and circulation. Pain or dysfunction of structures in or related to the abdomen may indicate a serious threat to physical health, may be a warning of impending pathologic processes or events, or may be an indication of emotional stress. Symptoms that have their primary source in the abdomen necessitate careful consideration, since critical emergencies sometimes involve complaints related to the abdomen or related structures. For example, a chief complaint of vomiting may in the final analysis be deemed associated with a mild case of the flu and not indicative of a serious threat to physical health. However, persistent or severe vomiting, even when associated with the flu, may precipitate a life-threatening imbalance of electrolytes and fluids and consequently result in cardiac dysrhythmias and death. Likewise, the patient in severe distress who complains of epigastric ''fullness,'' nausea, and diaphoresis may be experiencing symptoms as a result of any number of problems such as gastritis, an ulcer, a less serious problem, or a myocardial infarction. Triage professionals must consider the ''worst-case'' scenario for each patient so that a high index of suspicion can be maintained, ensuring that the patient's complaint receives a thorough analysis and the appropriate triage designation. Time can be a critical factor: delay may result in death in critical diagnoses such as a perforated ulcer. It is better for the triage professional to have an attitude that a critical problem must be disproved rather than to assume a patient is not in jeopardy until serious indications of a critical condition exist. This attitude is important in caring for elderly people, since they may not have classic signs and symptoms of critical problems. A strong knowledge base in pathophysiology of each body system is helpful in developing the ability to discriminate the best triage designation for each patient.

TRIAGE HISTORY

Much of the information obtained during completion of the general information section of the triage document relates directly to abdominal complaints and health. Further documentation related to general information should be added when the chief complaint involves the abdomen, rectum, or genitalia. For example, patients are asked what their weight is, or, if policy dictates or nursing judgment indicates, a weight is obtained by scale measurement. If the patient is a newborn, the nurse should inquire about the infant's birth weight. Remembering that a newborn commonly doubles its weight by 3 to 4 months of age and triples its birth weight by 1 year of age, the nurse quickly gains an understanding of the developmental appropriateness of the infant's growth. All patients with abdominal complaints should be asked about recent weight changes; the number of pounds or kilograms of change in the weight and the period within which the change occurred should be recorded on the triage record (Fig. 8–1). This information is particularly critical for infants, young children, and elderly persons because they are at higher risk for fluid disturbances since they are often unable to express thirst and their proportion of water to body mass differs from that of normal adults. Weight loss is also a significant indication of cancer or AIDS in some patients.

Nutrition is another important consideration to ask about in triage. When and what the patient last ate and drank and the specifics of the intake should be determined. For infants the triage nurse should determine whether they are breast-fed or bottle-fed and, if bottle-fed, the type of formula and whether it is fortified with iron. Ask whether the infant has a normal appetite, the number of ounces consumed or the duration of breast-feeding, and the number of hours between feedings. In children and adults it is helpful to determine nutritional intake to decide whether symptoms may be associated with inadequate intake or foods with a high risk for food poisoning. For patients with abdominal pain who may become candidates for surgery, food intake may be considered in determination of anesthesia risk and type of anesthesia used, so it is not too early to ask about intake in triage.

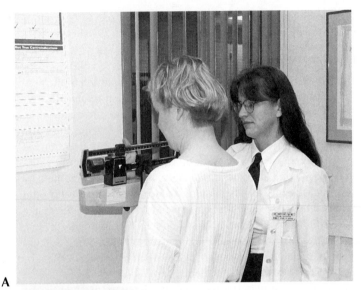

A

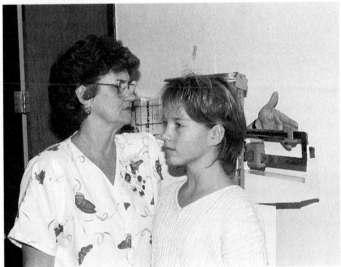

B

Fig. 8–1 **A,** All adult patients who are unsure of their weight or who report recent weight change should be weighed on a scale in triage. **B,** Pediatric patients should have a height/weight evaluation if growth appropriateness needs to be documented or if there are reports of recent weight changes.

In one segment of the general information section of the triage document all women are asked what the first day of their last menstrual period was and the number of pregnancies, live deliveries, stillbirths, tubal pregnancies, and spontaneous or therapeutic abortions they have had. If a woman has had a hysterectomy, the year and reason for the hysterectomy should be recorded. Obtaining the details of the reproductive history and prior procedures or surgeries involving the abdomen or related structures is helpful during the triage process, since scar tissue (internal adhesions), an increased risk for pregnancy complications, or an increased risk for recurrence of prior problems is possible. The triage nurse is only responsible for recording the patient's responses, not for judging the validity or reliability of responses, but when intuition "raises a warning flag" that a patient may be pregnant although she denies this possibility, the nurse should act on her/his intuition, particularly if there are serious ramifications for the woman or fetus.

PHYSICAL ASSESSMENT

During the history-taking process and physical assessment the triage nurse should carefully observe the patient's general appearance. Although appearances may be deceiving, the triage nurse can gain insight into the potential cause of the patient's distress by combining observations of the patient's general appearance with the history and physical assessment (Silen, 1991). Common problems of the abdomen and triage cues (many of which come from the general appearance) are listed in Box 8–1. Obtaining vital signs is a routine part of the physical assessment that the triage professional performs. If tympanic thermometers are used (Fig. 8–2) and fever is suspected but not verified by tympanic thermometer, an oral or rectal temperature should be obtained to confirm the accuracy of the temperature. Likewise, when patients appear febrile but have a normal oral temperature, the triage nurse should write a nursing order for emergency department (ED) personnel to obtain a rectal temperature. Rectal temperatures of infants may be obtained in triage if the physical setting allows (Fig. 8–3). If acetaminophen is used for alleviation of fever, the route of administration should be rectal if the patient needs to receive nothing by mouth or oral in the presence of diarrhea or vomiting or both.

| BOX 8–1 | **Causes of Abdominal Pain and Triage Cues** |

ABDOMINAL AORTIC ANEURYSM

Severe abdominal pain, pulsating mass (often not evident), hypotension; most common in elderly men who are smokers

APPENDICITIS

Cramping, burning, aching, colicky, dull, or gassy midabdominal pain; may radiate to other areas of abdomen; nausea, vomiting, diaphoresis, tachycardia, pallor, restlessness

ACUTE PANCREATITIS

Facial pallor, diaphoresis

ACUTE STRANGULATION OF GUT

Facial pallor, diaphoresis

ANEMIA

Pallor

BOWEL OBSTRUCTION

Sunken cheeks, hollow eyes

CHOLECYSTITIS

Cramping, burning, aching, dull, or gassy right-side upper-quadrant midabdominal pain; may radiate to other areas of abdomen; nausea, vomiting, diaphoresis, tachycardia, pallor, restlessness; most often occurs between 10 P.M. and 2 A.M.

CONSTIPATION

Change in patient's normal evacuation pattern; abdominal discomfort; bloating

DIARRHEA

EMOTIONAL STRESS

INTESTINAL OBSTRUCTION

Cramping, burning, aching, colicky, dull, or gassy midabdominal pain; may radiate to other areas of abdomen; nausea, vomiting, diaphoresis, tachycardia, pallor, restlessness

| BOX 8–1 | ## Causes of Abdominal Pain and Triage Cues—cont'd |

INTUSSUSCEPTION

Repeated screaming attacks, legs drawn up; restlessness; diminished feeding or appetite; vomiting, jellylike red stool, fever, abdominal distention

PANCREATITIS

Severe upper-quadrant abdominal pain with referral to back, worse when lying down, accompanied by nausea and vomiting

PERFORATED GASTRIC ULCER

Facial pallor, diaphoresis

PERITONITIS

Restlessness, knees drawn up for comfort; steady, aching pain increased by movement

RUPTURED OVARIAN CYST

Sudden pain often associated with exercise or intercourse, usually unilateral

RUPTURED TUBAL PREGNANCY

Deathly pallor, gasping respirations

THORACIC EMERGENCIES

Nasal flaring

TOXEMIA

Dull gaze of eyes, ashen skin color

URINARY TRACT INFECTION

Dysuria, frequent urination, abdominal discomfort, flank pain

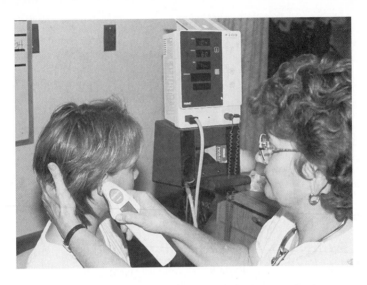

Fig. 8–2 Tympanic temperature assessment is rapid. The tympanic thermometer should be aimed toward the child's face and must fit well in the ear canal.

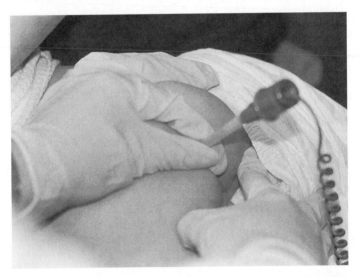

Fig. 8–3 Taking the rectal temperature is the most accurate method of temperature assessment in pediatric patients younger than 3 years old.

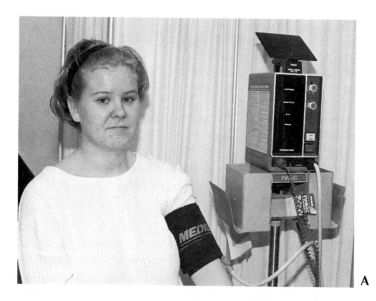

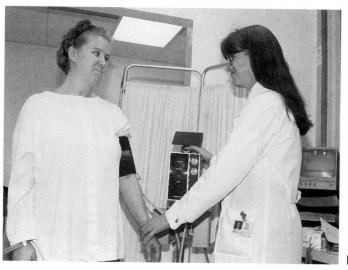

Fig. 8–4 **A,** The triage nurse evaluates blood pressure and pulse in both sitting and standing positions for orthostatic changes. Evaluation of the patient's general appearance is concurrent. **B,** When the patient stands during orthostatic assessment, the triage nurse also evaluates the patient for dizziness, nausea, and pallor.

Orthostatic vital signs should be obtained in all patients with a chief complaint related to the abdomen or female reproductive organs, to assess the patient's state of circulatory homeostasis. The patient's tolerance of position changes during assessment of orthostatic vital signs should also be recorded, that is, whether the patient tolerated the position changes well, became light-headed, or was unable to tolerate the entire series in the assessment of orthostatic vital signs (Fig. 8–4). A patient with tachycardia or hypotension at rest should be triaged as emergent or immediate, regardless of the chief complaint. A common cause of fluid volume depletion is inadequate fluid intake to meet the body's demands. Fluid volume depletion is often identified during orthostatic vital sign assessment. The triage nurse should be aware that patients at particularly high risk include the very young, the elderly, the disabled, and those with certain diseases such as cystic fibrosis. Children with cystic fibrosis may underestimate their fluid needs and are more likely to become dehydrated, particularly during hot weather and with exercise (Bar et al., 1992).

ABDOMINAL PAIN

As is true of thoracic pain, abdominal pain occurs for many reasons. Because of the characteristic causes of abdominal pain, it is helpful for the triage professional to obtain as clear a description of the abdominal pain as possible (Box 8–2). Allowing the patients to express the quality and characteristics of their pain without interruption is important in obtaining an objective report and making a reliable triage decision. The triage professional also must interview patients about the timing, onset, and remedies relevant to the pain. Obtaining information about prior episodes and related diagnoses associated with abdominal health is necessary for a complete picture of the patient's presentation. If the patient is extremely uncomfortable and cannot volunteer information when presented with open-ended questions, the nurse, using the framework for analyzing a symptom, should ask closed-ended questions, providing examples of answers if necessary.

Discomfort alone, even when extreme, should not be cause for emergent or immediate triage designation unless the patient, by history and physical presentation, has a problem that is char-

BOX 8–2	**Key Questions To Ask Patients With Abdominal Pain**

GENERAL, OPEN-ENDED QUESTIONS EVERYONE SHOULD BE ASKED

- When did your abdominal pain start?
- Do you remember what you were doing when the pain first started?
- Did your discomfort come on suddenly or gradually?
- Do you have any ideas about what may have brought on your abdominal pain?
- Can you describe your discomfort specifically—how it felt when it first came on and how it feels now?
- Please point to where your discomfort is worst.
- Does your discomfort radiate? (Ask about flank, legs, and shoulders.)
- On a scale of 1 to 10, with 10 being the worst pain you've ever felt or imagined, how would you rate your pain at this moment? When it began? After you tried to alleviate it?
- Do you have any other symptoms? (nausea, vomiting, diaphoresis, dizziness)
- Have you done anything to try to make the pain go away, including using any home remedies, nonprescription medications, or prescribed medications or treatments?
- Do you have a history of abdominal pain? Have you called your primary health care provider about your pain today?
- Are you under treatment for any health problems?
- Have you ever had abdominal surgery or surgical procedures that involve your abdomen?

SPECIFIC, CLOSED-ENDED QUESTIONS THAT MAY BE HELPFUL

- When did you last urinate?
- Have you had burning, increased frequency of urination, hesitancy (you can urinate only a little even though you feel you have to urinate very urgently), or a change in the color or odor of your urine?
- When was your last bowel movement?
- Was there any change in the color, shape, consistency, or appearance of the stool?
- Have you vomited or had diarrhea today? If so, how many times, and what did it look like?

Continued.

| BOX 8–2 | **Key Questions To Ask Patients With Abdominal Pain—cont'd** |

- Do you feel that there is any association between your gastrointestinal or urinary symptoms and your discomfort?
- Have you experienced any abdominal trauma today or in the past?
- Do you think there is any chance that you may have a sexually transmissible disease? Do you have any discharge from your genital area?
- Do you think there is any chance you may be pregnant? What was the first day of your last menstrual period?
- Do you think there may be an association between your pain and your menstrual cycle?

acteristically emergent, for example, abdominal aortic aneurysm. In addition to asking routine questions about the time and manner of onset, specific questions should be asked about common causes of abdominal pain (Box 8–2). It is difficult to diagnose causes of abdominal pain in children, and it may be difficult to triage correctly children who arrive at triage with abdominal pain. The triage nurse should err on the side of caution when triaging children with abdominal pain, since a high morbidity rate is associated with perforation of the appendix in children (Dolgin et al., 1992). Although abdominal pain has rarely been a symptom of hypertensive crisis in children, because of this possibility and because it is helpful to observe blood pressure, blood pressure should be measured in all children with abdominal discomfort (Van-Why et al., 1993). In infants with abdominal pain (suspected because of knee withdrawal, grimacing, and relentless crying), any stools should be saved to be evaluated for the presence of blood; this is a particularly valuable discovery when intussusception is the cause of pain, since this problem may cause death when it is not recognized and treated early (Stringer et al., 1992).

The triage nurse can develop ideas about the origin of abdominal pain based on the characteristics used to describe the pain. Understanding the possible origin of the patient's pain is helpful in determining the level of acuity assigned in triage.

Visceral pain that emanates from the abdominal organs is usually diffuse and intermittent, and the specific location difficult to identify. Often it is felt at differing levels at the midline of the abdomen. Visceral pain is usually described as cramping, burning, aching, colicky, dull, or gassy and is often accompanied by nausea, vomiting, diaphoresis, tachycardia, pallor, and restlessness. Causes of visceral pain include appendicitis, cholecystitis, and intestinal obstruction. Parietal pain develops subsequent to visceral pain and is caused by peritoneal inflammation. Parietal pain is usually a persistent, aching pain that is severe and aggravated by movement. Sometimes abdominal pain is referred from other parts of the body, most often from organs innervated from the same region of the spinal cord feeding the abdomen. The triage nurse must take all likely possibilities of abdominal pain into account when determining acuity level (Jess, 1993). Common patterns of referred pain are listed in Box 8–3.

Discerning the presence of immediate or relatively recent

BOX 8–3	**Common Patterns of Referred Abdominal Pain**

SITE	**REFERRING VISCUS**
Left shoulder	Left diaphragmatic irritation (spleen, subphrenic fluid or abscess), esophagus, heart
Right shoulder	Right diaphragmatic irritation, liver
Epigastrium	Stomach, transverse colon
Right upper quadrant of abdomen	Liver, biliary tree, pylorus, duodenum
Flank	Kidney, pancreas
Sacrum, lumbar area	Uterus, rectum
Hypogastrium	Colon, kidney
Groin, genitalia	Ureter, bladder
Umbilicus	Appendix, midgut

From Yamada T et al: *Textbook of gastroenterology,* vols 1 and 2, 1991, Lippincott.

abdominal trauma is important. As in all traumatic injuries, if a trauma has occurred the nurse must learn about the circumstances of the traumatic injury (Box 8–4). It is important to remember that patients with abdominal trauma may also have damage to retroperitoneal structures such as the kidneys. Patients should be queried about the presence of hematuria. Gross hematuria is a significant indicator that the patient's triage designation should be emergent, since this finding is strongly correlated with shock and significant injury for both urologic and extrarenal abdominal organs (Knudson et al., 1992).

Patients with hematuria in the absence of abdominal trauma should be asked about signs and symptoms of infection, presence of congenital abnormalities of the urinary system, history of renal calculi, cancer, or drug use, and exercise. Hematuria is a common problem in children and is often benign (Neiberger, 1994). In any individual, signifiers that the problem is immediate include abdominal trauma, indication by general appearance, severe discomfort, and changes in orthostatic vital signs.

Learning about the menstrual history of women and past abdominal procedures or surgeries is important. Determining the normalcy of bowel and bladder function is critical. Changes from the usual pattern and appearance of urine and feces are of particular importance, since ''normal'' is a relative term for each individual. When asking about bowel function, the nurse can quickly determine the most recent bowel movement, the color and consistency of stool, and whether the patient notices

---

| BOX 8–4 | **Facts To Be Determined in Triage of Patients With Abdominal Trauma** |

- Circumstances of trauma
- Whether trauma was blunt or sharp
- What object was involved in trauma
- Velocity of patient or object or both at time of trauma
- Sequelae at time of injury (loss of consciousness and associated injuries)
- Last ingestion of food or fluid

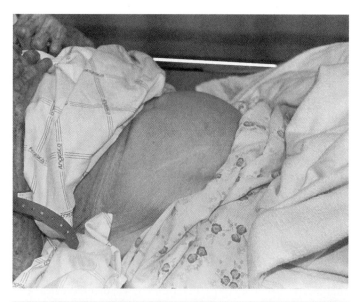

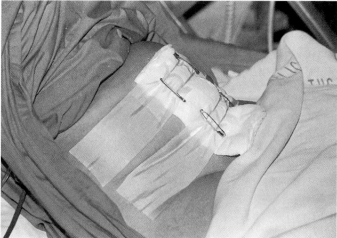

Fig. 8–5 Abdominal distention often accompanies bowel obstruction.

changes from the usual presentation or pattern. The patient should also be asked about the urine function, specifically, about the frequency, amount, color, and characteristics of the urine. If the patient reports a change in bowel or bladder function, the changes should be recorded concisely. A patient who has diarrhea or vomiting should be asked about the number of episodes in the last 24 hours, as well as the pattern of time and frequency since symptom onset. Patients who report having diarrhea should be asked whether they had constipation before the onset of diarrhea, since one of the most frequent causes of diarrhea is constipation in the patient with bowel obstruction, a common problem in elderly individuals (Fig. 8–5). In addition to considering changes in bowel or bladder function as incitants to or concurrent with abdominal discomfort, the triage professional should specifically consider other precipitating factors and the patient should be asked about specific factors that may have caused the onset of abdominal pain, when these are suspected.

In women with abdominal pain who may have a history or presentation of pelvic inflammatory disease or in men with a chief complaint of needing ''an all-over check'' or ''penile discharge'' on arrival at triage, determining whether there has been a recent change in sexual partner or whether there has been vaginal or penile discharge should be considered important.

Individuals who have renal calculi often arrive at triage with a chief complaint of abdominal pain, which may originate in or radiate to the flank area. A patient who has a self-reported or confirmed history of renal calculi is normally triaged as emergent or immediate, since the severity of pain associated with renal calculi is comparable only to childbirth or myocardial infarction in degree of discomfort. In triage a urine sample should be requested of the patient if possible, to observe for hematuria and to obtain a sample to be strained for calculi. The patient who is unable to provide a urine sample should be told to inform personnel when providing a sample is possible, and should be informed that all urine must be strained from the time of triage until discharge from the hospital.

Often it is possible to increase one's index of suspicion for a problem based on the patient's prior history of problems, demographics, and the quality of the patient's discomfort. Pain that is crampy, intermittently severe, and located in the upper right quadrant of the abdomen, for example, may be associated with cholecystitis. Patients should be specifically asked to describe the nature and location of discomfort at the time of presentation and since the onset of the pain (Fig. 8–6). Patients should be specifically asked about radiation of pain to the shoulders (positive Kehr's sign), since this may indicate intrabdominal bleeding, thereby cueing the examiner to the need for emergent triage designation. Severity of a patient's pain should be determined using the severity scale for subjective pain for the time of onset, for the present severity, and for the severity following any palliative treatments or medications used at home.

Patients with abdominal pain must be specifically asked about the use of palliative treatments and medications. They must be asked whether they have used nonprescription remedies such as bismuth solutions, cathartics, and antacids, home rem-

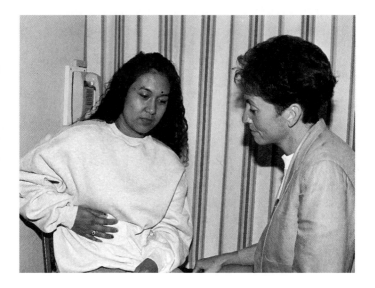

Fig. 8–6   The patient should be asked to identify the location of abdominal pain. Right upper quadrant pain is common in cholecystitis.

edies such as baking soda or cola drinks, prescribed medications such as pain relievers or acid inhibitors, or therapies such as a heating pad, massage, or enemas. It is important to ask about palliatives not only to determine their effectiveness in relieving the patient's discomfort, but also to consider their effect as potential precipitating factors of the patient's chief complaint and to be aware of their effect on other diagnoses or therapeutics specific to the patient. When a patient with abdominal pain has a history of abdominal pain and prior associated diagnoses, it is important to ask whether the patient's current discomfort is similar to or different from episodes of pain associated with chronic or past medical problems. It is also necessary, particularly in the current climate of insurance issues in health care, to determine whether the patient has sought medical care for the presenting symptoms within 24 hours before the ED visit or whether the patient has called her/his primary health care provider since the onset of the abdominal pain.

It is important to consider demographics while observing the patient and listening to the history and during the brief physical assessment performed in triage. Understanding the high-risk populations for a variety of problems related to abdominal pain is also helpful in determining the appropriate triage category for the patient. For example, children may have abdominal pain in association with emotional stress, appendicitis (early or late), or constipation and more rarely, in association with life-threatening problems such as intussusception of the bowel. Adolescents have abdominal pain in association with emotional stress, appendicitis, constipation, Mittelschmerz or endometriosis (girls), sexually transmitted diseases (particularly chlamydial diseases and gonorrhea), and more serious, life-threatening problems such as leukemia. Older adults may have abdominal pain as a result of constipation, diverticulitis, appendicitis, cholecystitis, or more life-threatening problems such as bowel obstruction, infarcted bowel, or gastrointestinal bleeding. These examples are not meant to imply that certain problems related to the abdomen are found only in age-related populations, but to explicate that there is a higher index of suspicion for certain problems within age-related populations. Of course, many problems are quite common, particularly in adults, and are considered as possibilities depending on the patient's presentation. When a problem is considered highly likely, the patient is triaged accordingly (Fig. 8–7).

Ethnicity is also relevant when considering potential causes of abdominal pain. For example, Mexican patients, particularly women, have a higher rate of cholecystitis than the general population. Japanese patients have a higher rate of stomach cancer than the general population. Native Americans have a higher incidence of gastrointestinal bleeding.

Physical assessment in triage of the patient with discomfort in the abdominal or a related area is limited by the area of involvement (Box 8–5). In addition to normal vital sign measurement it is important to assess orthostatic blood pressure and pulse, even if only to compare the patient's sitting and standing vital signs. Accurate assessment of the patient's temperature is important in determining the presence of fever and fever-related causes such as appendicitis or flu.

Performance of techniques other than observation of the abdomen is not generally practical in the triage area, although

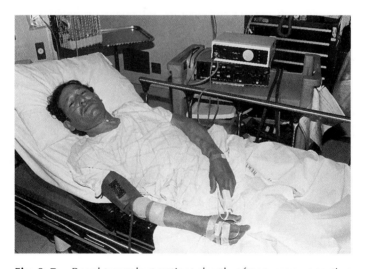

Fig. 8–7   Renal transplant patient shortly after surgery reporting to triage is designated emergent status after evaluation of general appearance, brief history, physical assessment, and objective data gathering.

BOX 8–5	Physical Assessment of Patients With Abdominal Pain

- Measurement of orthostatic vital signs
- Accurate assessment of temperature
- Observation for abdominal distention
- Assessment of whether abdomen is soft or firm
- Assessment for abdominal tenderness

the nurse may be able to inquire about and assess for softness of firmness of the abdomen. When an abdomen is "hard," it should then be determined by history whether this condition is chronic or new since it may be associated with muscular tone in some individuals. The "worst-case" scenario is that a severely painful, distended, and firm abdomen is indicative of a "surgical" abdomen in an acutely ill person. Even in the absence of orthostatic vital sign changes the patient should be triaged as emergent or immediate, since complications may be avoided with prompt and appropriate medical evaluation and treatment.

Treatment of individuals in triage who arrive with abdominal pain is consistent with that of any person with pain or discomfort (Box 8–6). Dealing with the patient in a calm manner, teaching relaxation breathing, offering a cool cloth for the face and a container for emesis if nausea or vomiting is a problem are all helpful actions. The individual and significant others who are present with the patient should be informed that the patient will be on a strict regimen of receiving nothing by mouth until seen and treated by ED personnel. If the patient has hypotension or significant orthostatic vital sign changes, every effort should be made to provide the patient with a gurney or bed to lie on for safety and comfort. In addition, patients who are vomiting frequently should be placed in an area out of contact with the general population, since the sound of retching and vomiting causes many people to have a sympathetic response.

If the patient reports having vomited at home or vomits in triage and direct observation and guaiac testing of the emesis are possible, evaluation for hematemesis is important. Re-

BOX 8–6	**Triage Treatment of Patients With Abdominal Pain**

- Rest
- Emesis basin
- Cool cloth for face
- Regimen of nothing by mouth
- Encouragement of relaxation breathing
- Position of comfort
- Education regarding bathroom facilities
- Instruction, if sample of feces or urine is needed
- Education regarding need to delay administration of pain relief agents until examination

member to take into account dietary and pharmaceutical factors that can affect the accuracy of guaiac testing.

ABDOMINAL DISTENTION

Observing the abdomen for distention is helpful but limited, since the abdomen is not visualized with the patient in the supine position, unless the patient is an infant or toddler. If the patient has an obviously distended abdomen, the degree to which this is important varies according to the patient's history and remaining assessment data. Common causes of abdominal distention are listed in Box 8–7.

Further assessment data should be collected or requested according to the triage professional's index of suspicion for various causes of distention. For example, although some women report normal menstrual periods and deny the possibility of pregnancy, obvious distention and an intuitive sense a nurse has that the patient may be pregnant lead to a nurse's order for measurement of fetal heart tones or a rapid urine pregnancy test, if the policies of the ED allow. Even if a triage professional can note only the presence of distention, it is important to record this observation, since ED personnel can then be sure to inspect, auscultate, percuss, and palpate the abdomen with careful attention to detail and results. Critical findings associated with high mortality and morbidity rates are given in Box 8–8.

BOX 8–7	**Six Common Causes of Abdominal Distention: The Six Fs**

- Fat
- Fetus
- Fluid
- Flatus
- Feces
- Fatal or fibroid tumor

BOX 8–8	**Critical Findings in Evaluation of Abdominal Pain That Cue Immediate Triage Designation**

- Orthostatic vital sign changes >20 beats/min (systolic blood pressure or pulse)
- Absence of femoral pulses
- Pulsatile mass obvious on inspection of the abdomen
- Major abdominal trauma
- Fever >102° F with obvious distress
- Severe pain with hematuria or history of renal calculi
- Severe pain with firm or distended abdomen
- Epigastric pain with hematemesis or history of gastrointestinal bleeding

---

Patients with a chief complaint of abdominal distention often have other symptoms that are of equal concern to the patient such as urinary retention, cancer affecting the contents of the abdomen, fecal impaction and constipation, or flatus. If the patient is unable to give a clear history because of aphasia, developmental disability, or other factors influencing communication, the triage nurse should determine the time and manner of onset of the abdominal distention. If the abdomen, in addition to being distended, is tender, painful, and firm, the patient should be triaged as emergent, since the cause of the distention should be discerned without delay. Causes such as urinary retention or peritoneal inflammation may lead to critical problems if they are not diagnosed and treated quickly.

When infants arrive at triage with abdominal distention, it is important to ask about the infant's feeding type and pattern. Additives to formula, such as iron, should be inquired about. When evaporated milk is used, preparation and concentration of the milk should be determined, as well as the presence of commonly used additives such as corn syrup. If the infant is homeless or lives in transient conditions, it is necessary to determine what type of water the infant ingests, to understand the risk of infection that may exist if unhealthful water is used. When infants are breast-fed, the duration and intervals of breast-feeding should be determined, as well as changes in the timing or pattern of feeding and changes in the mother's diet. The potential for abdominal distention because of lactose intolerance is high for black or dark-skinned infants and children who have a clear association of distention following the ingestion of dairy products.

INTRACTABLE DIARRHEA

Diarrhea can cause life-threatening dehydration and an imbalance of electrolytes that may lead to dysrhythmias and death. Elderly and pediatric patients in particular are at high risk for fluid and electrolyte imbalance and need careful evaluation for appropriate triage. Important questions to ask during the triage history should include questions about travel, change in dietary habits, and whether the patient has acquired immunodeficiency syndrome (AIDS). Determining the number of episodes of diarrhea before arrival at triage is important in evaluating the likelihood of complications of diarrhea. The consistency, odor, and amount of fluid expelled with diarrhea are critical information. If the patient is able to provide a stool specimen, it should be used for guaiac testing and laboratory analysis, if later requested by the physician. Blood or mucus in the stool, increased frequency of bowel movements, abdominal pain, and fever are common in individuals with shigellosis (Mathan and Mathan, 1991). Individuals at high risk for infectious diarrhea include those who have travelled to developing nations or in areas where water may not be clean, those consuming unusual foods at restaurants, banquets, or social events, those with AIDS, children in day care, and those in institutions (Yamada et al., 1991). Diarrhea is the most common gastrointestinal problem in patients with AIDS; approximately half of all patients with human immunodeficiency virus (HIV) will have diarrhea. Characteristic diarrhea in patients with AIDS is nonbloody and watery. It may be accompanied by weight loss and malnutrition. Causes of diarrhea in patients with AIDS include infections and medications (Anastasi, 1993).

Prior problems with constipation should be noted, since diarrhea preceded by constipation is a common presentation in bowel obstruction, a critical surgical emergency.

Physical assessment of individuals with intractable diarrhea should include observation of oral mucous membranes for moisture and general inspection of the face for signs of dehydration such as sunken eyes, pallor, and lethargy. In children examination of the fontanelle is helpful. Orthostatic vital signs should be assessed if the individual is tachycardic or complains of dizziness on standing or extreme fatigue. Individuals who exhibit signs of serious dehydration (e.g., tachycardia >120 beats/min, or orthostatic vital sign changes) should be triaged as emergent.

Patients who have incontinent diarrhea should be provided with a bathroom and materials for cleaning themselves, with assistance as needed. A private waiting area and diapers should be provided if the patient is not emergent and waiting is required. Significant others should be provided with gloves if they are assisting the patient, since they are likely to come into contact with the patient's body fluids.

VOMITING

Vomiting may be a symptom associated with a chief complaint or it may be the chief complaint of a patient seeking emergency services. The nature of the emesis should be determined immediately, to rule out the possibility of gastrointestinal bleeding. The patient should specifically be asked about the presence of ''coffee-ground'' flecks or particles in the emesis or the presence of frank blood. The number of episodes of hematemesis and amount of emesis should be determined. Patients with suspected gastrointestinal bleeding should be triaged as emergent. Some patients report specks of frank blood after many episodes of vomiting, a presentation more characteristic of tract irritation than of acute gastrointestinal bleeding. Unless these patients have a history of gastrointestinal bleeding or are considered at high risk because of risk factors such as chronic alcoholism or persistent use of nonsteroidal antiinflammatory drugs or anticoagulants, they may be triaged safely as urgent.

As with intractable diarrhea, patients with persistent vomiting are at risk for dehydration and consequent complications. Patients with hyperemesis and gravidity are at risk not only for dehydration but also for spontaneous abortion if they have persistent fluid and electrolyte depletion. In addition to evaluating the patient with hyperemesis and gravidity for dehydration, the triage professional should write a nursing order for measurement of fetal heart tones, to be evaluated once the patient is in the ED. During the interview process this patient should be asked about fetal movement, particularly if she is more than 16 weeks pregnant. Some ED policies indicate that patients who are more than 20 weeks must be seen in the obstetric department for evaluation and triaged back to the ED once it has been determined that the fetus is not in danger and the pregnancy is not threatened.

All patients with vomiting should be placed on a regimen of receiving nothing by mouth until physician clearance has been obtained. Infants and children with intractable diarrhea or persistent vomiting need frequent reassessment in triage if entry into the ED is delayed, since they are at high risk for dehydration complications. A physician order should be obtained for oral administration of an electrolyte-rich fluid in infants, if appropriate, during the waiting period before medical evaluation and treatment are available.

All patients with persistent vomiting and intractable diarrhea should be weighed on a scale, and a record should be made of recent weight change, birth weight in newborns and young infants, and usual weight in children and adults.

All individuals on a routine regimen of medications should be specifically queried about their last dose and the time frame wherein medication absorption may have been affected by the gastrointestinal symptoms, and this information should be highlighted on the triage record. Likewise, if an accidental or intentional medication or drug overdose is suspected (which may be responsible for gastrointestinal symptoms), the reason for this suspicion should be concisely recorded. When overdose is a potential problem, the patient should be triaged as emergent. Communication with personnel is critical in ensuring patient safety if patients are considered at risk for harming themselves. (For further discussion on this subject see Chapter 12.)

RECTAL PAIN

Rectal pain can be uncomfortable and distressing. It is important to question patients who arrive at triage with this chief complaint about common causes of rectal pain such as anxiety and hemorrhoids. They should also be asked about noticeable physical changes in the rectum (e.g., rectal prolapse). Patients may volunteer information regarding the association between the introduction of foreign objects into the rectum and the onset of rectal pain. Such patients should be queried about the continued presence of the object; if it was removed, they should be asked whether the removal was physically traumatic. If the object is a vibrator and it continues to oscillate in the bowel, the patient should be triaged immediately for an emergent surgical evaluation. It is also important that any patient with a history associated with sexual and social significance be treated with confidentiality and dignity. Patients may have foreign objects in the rectum as a result of digestive passage, for example, a chicken bone. This is a prevalent problem in individuals who wear dentures (Davis, 1991). Patients, often prisoners, may hide drugs in the anal canal; concern for container rupture must also exist.

In addition to the analysis of answers to questions about symptoms, which are asked of all patients, patients with rectal pain should be asked about rectal discharge. If they report rectal bleeding, the color and amount of the blood should be recorded.

GENITAL PAIN

Causes of genital pain vary according to the gender of the patient. Patients of both sexes may have genital pain in the presence of a direct hernia. When questioned about anatomic changes, patients often report a local bulge. Physical assessment is, of course, not possible in the triage area unless the triage setting is private or the patient is an infant.

Women who report genital pain should be queried about precipitating factors, including the types of soaps and feminine products used and accidental traumatic injuries. The triage nurse should not assume, even in children, that complaints of vulvar inflammation or vaginitis are certain indicators of sexual abuse. Although the triage nurse should be alert to the possibility of sexual abuse, the majority of complaints of vulvar inflammation and secondary vaginitis are benign (Aruda, 1992).

Any patient with rectal or sexual trauma associated with sexual assault should be triaged directly into the ED that treats victims of sexual abuse. Many EDs have a team of professionals who are on call for the evaluation of victims of sexual assault. These specially trained team members interview and examine the patient, collect samples from the patient for forensic purposes, and ensure emotional support of the patient. Some EDs however, particularly those in rural areas or small EDs, may not have a specialized team, and it is important to be familiar with what information must be collected during the triage process. Because of the psychologic trauma associated with reporting a sexual assault, the patient should be interviewed in a quiet, private setting. The vital information to be gleaned during the interview process, which is relevant for both male and female victims of sexual trauma, is outlined in Box 8–9.

If, because the historian is unreliable, the triage professional is unable to determine whether the patient should be triaged into the system for sexual abuse victims, consultation with the charge nurse and physician should take place in order to make the right decision for the patient. This is particularly critical when the patient is an infant or child, since these patients are usually unable to provide clear historical information. Childhood sexual abuse is a common problem; one national survey indicated that 27% of women and 16% of men have been sexually abused as children (Gibbons and Vincent, 1994). For this reason the triage nurse and all health professionals must be familiar with indications of this problem. One of the most accurate indicators of sexual abuse is disclosure by the child. If there is any disclosure by a child that the child has been abused, the triage nurse must record the child's statement and see that the child is interviewed and examined specifically for this problem by professionals assigned to this area (Dubowitz et al.,

| BOX 8–9 | **Critical Information To Be Obtained During Triage Interview of Victims of Sexual Assault** |

I. History of the event.
  A. Time, date and place.
  B. Use of force, threats of force, and the like.
    1. Type of violence used.
    2. Threats of violence.
    3. Use of restraints.
    4. Number of assailants.
    5. Use of alcohol or drugs.
    6. Loss of consciousness.
  C. Type of assault.
    1. Fondling.
    2. Vaginal penetration or attempted penetration.
    3. Oral penetration or attempted penetration.
    4. Anal penetration or attempted penetration.
    5. Ejaculation on or in body? Where?
    6. Condom used?
II. Gynecologic history (some points optional).
  A. Use of birth control before attack. (Any missed pills?)
  B. Last normal menstrual period.
  C. Last voluntary intercourse (within past week).
  D. Gravidity and parity.
  E. Recent gynecologic surgery.
  F. History of recent sexually transmitted disease.
III. Medical history.
  A. Current medications.
  B. Tetanus immunization status.
  C. Allergies.
  D. Douching, bathing, urination, or defecation following rape.

From Rosen P, ed: *Emergency medicine: concepts and clinical practice,* ed 3, 3 vols, St Louis, 1993, Mosby.

1992). The triage nurse should also be concerned about the potential for sexual abuse in girls who arrive at triage with a chief complaint of vaginal foreign body, since this may be an indicator of sexual abuse (Herman, 1994).

Not all children who are sexually abused have classic signs and symptoms of abuse. Some individuals have an intuitive sense of children who are experiencing serious psychologic and physical trauma but who are not being seen in the ED for a related reason. Triage nurses should not feel embarrassed about sharing their concerns. Signs that sexual abuse may be occurring include posttraumatic stress disorder, attention-deficit hyperactivity disorder, secondary enuresis and encopresis, nightmares, and inappropriate sexual behavior. Furthermore, it is known that children express themselves most easily through nonverbal communication, often in the waiting room or another neutral place (Elliott and Peterson, 1993).

Patients with dyspareunia and postcoital bleeding should be treated in the ED, since this presentation may be indicative of cervical cancer. Dyspareunia may also indicate that the patient has had intercourse with a partner who has a large penis that her vagina can easily accommodate without trauma.

Male patients who arrive at triage with genital pain should be queried about the specific location of the pain and association of the pain with trauma. When serious problems, such as testicular torsion, are suspected, it is crucial that the patient be triaged as emergent. Testicular torsion occurs in 1 of 160 men 25 years of age or younger. It must be recognized early to maintain a high salvage rate (100% if correction occurs within 3 hours, but only 10% to 20% if correction occurs within 10 to 24 hours) (Prater and Overdorf, 1991). Acute scrotal pain with associated nausea and vomiting are hallmarks of testicular torsion. Questions about sexual activity and contraceptive products that may be irritating or may cause an allergic response may be saved until the patient is in a more confidential setting but must be included in the interview process.

Pain in the genitalia that is chronic or is likely to be associated with sexually transmissible diseases may enable the triage professional to designate the patient as ''nonurgent.'' Some hospitals may have a policy that requires referral of patients with complaints of sexually transmissible disease to a clinic for the treatment of such diseases. If the patient is not going to be seen on the day of arrival at triage, giving the patient brief but specific information regarding the use of condoms or avoidance of membrane contact with possibly infected genitalia is important, to avoid the continued spread of the sexually transmissible disease.

The presence or recent use of foreign objects or sexual aids involving the genitalia should be assessed, if relevant, and the information recorded accordingly.

VAGINAL BLEEDING

Patients with vaginal bleeding must have the immediacy of their condition determined swiftly in order to be triaged for comfort and safety (Box 8–10). During the history the triage nurse should determine the severity of the bleeding by asking the patient how many pads or tampons the patient is saturating each hour or day. The symptom analysis should also include questions regarding the color of the blood and whether there is an association of the amount of bleeding with position change or activity. It is necessary to determine the presence or likelihood of pregnancy, the date of the last menstrual period, and a history of gynecologic procedures or diagnoses. Antepartum patients who are more than 20 weeks pregnant may be triaged directly to obstetric care if ED policies so indicate. Postpartum patients with excessive vaginal bleeding should be triaged immediately, since the risk of fluid deficit and complications such as incomplete expulsion of the placenta exist. Antepartum patients who have signs and symptoms of impending spontaneous abortion should be triaged immediately to avoid fetal expulsion in the waiting area and because these patients usually have emotional distress and pain, whether loudly expressed or not.

Patients who have a chief complaint of vaginal bleeding who do not have critical problems with vital signs, suspected pregnancy-associated problems, or excessive vaginal bleeding may be triaged as "nonurgent" or "urgent," depending on the overall presentation of the patient, resources for nonurgent care if the patient should be triaged for clinical or primary care services, and policies of the department responsible for assessing

BOX 8–10	**Vaginal Bleeding That Necessitates Immediate Triage Designation**

- Saturation of more than one pad or tampon per hour
- Orthostatic hypotension or tachycardia or both
- Bright red bleeding with pregnancy of more than 16 weeks
- Symptoms of impending spontaneous abortion

| BOX 8–11 | **Risk Factors for Ectopic Pregnancy Relevant to Triage** |

- Sexually transmitted disease or pelvic infection
- Progesterone-only contraception
- Previous surgery for ectopic pregnancy
- Tubal surgery
- Induced abortion
- Intrauterine device
- Tubal sterilization
- Endometriosis
- Maternal cigarette smoking
- Oral contraceptives and intrauterine device at time of conception

the patient in triage. The triage nurse must be alert to the possibility of ectopic pregnancy if the patient has abdominal pain, amenorrhea, and vaginal bleeding. One in 12 of all first-trimester complications of pregnancy was an ectopic pregnancy in one published study (Norman, 1991), and a 4.5-fold increase of ectopic pregnancies has been seen in the United States since 1970 (although the mortality rate has decreased by 90%) (Ory, 1992). Knowledge of the patient's risk factors for ectopic pregnancy may also be helpful (Box 8–11), although all women of childbearing age who complain of abdominal pain or abnormal bleeding should be considered at possible risk for ectopic pregnancy (Benrubi, 1994). Women who smoke are at much higher risk for ectopic pregnancies, and the risk increases with the number of cigarettes smoked (Coste et al., 1991).

REFERENCES

Anastasi J: AIDS update: caring for patients with diarrhea, *Nursing* 23(8):68, 1993.

Aruda M: Vulvovaginitis in the prepubertal child, *Nurse Pract Forum* 3(3):149, 1992.

Bar O et al: Voluntary dehydration and heat intolerance in cystic fibrosis, *Lancet* 339(8795):696, 1992.

Benrubi G: *Obstetric and gynecologic emergencies,* 1994, Lippincott.

Coste J, Job-Spira, Fernandez H: Increased risk of ectopic pregnancy with maternal cigarette smoking, *Am J Public Health* 81(2):199, 1991.

Davis D: A chicken bone in the rectum, *Arch Emerg Med* 8(1):62, 1991.

Dolgin S, Beck A, Tartter P: The risk of perforation when children with possible appendicitis are observed in the hospital, *Surg Gynecol Obstet* 175(4):320, 1992.

Dubowitz H, Black M, Harrington D: The diagnosis of child sexual abuse, *Am J Dis Child* 146(6):688, 1992.

Elliott A, Peterson L: Maternal sexual abuse of male children: when to suspect and how to uncover it, *Postgrad Med* 94(1):169, 175, 180, 1993.

Gibbons M, Vincent E: Childhood sexual abuse, *Am Fam Physician* 49(1):125, 1994.

Herman G: Vaginal foreign bodies and child sexual abuse, *Arch Pediatr Adolesc Med* 148(2):195, 1994.

Jess L: Acute abdominal pain: revealing the source, *Nursing* 34, 1993.

Knudson M et al: Hematuria as a predictor of abdominal injury after blunt trauma, *Am J Surg* 164(5):482, 1992.

Mathan V, Mathan M: Intestinal manifestations of invasive diarrheas and their diagnosis, *Rev Infect Dis* 13(suppl 4):s311, 1991.

Neiberger R: The ABCs of evaluating children with hematuria, *Am Fam Physician* 49(3):623, 1994.

Norman S: An audit of the management of ectopic pregnancy, *Br J Obstet Gynaecol* 98(12):1267, 1991.

Ory S: New options for diagnosis and treatment of ectopic pregnancy, *JAMA* 267(4):534, 1992.

Prater J, Overdorf B: Testicular torsion: a surgical emergency, *Am Fam Physician* 44(3):834, 1991.

Rosen P, ed: *Emergency medicine: concepts and clinical practice,* ed 3, 3 vols, St Louis, 1992, Mosby.

Silen W: *Cope's early diagnosis of the acute abdomen,* ed 18, New York, 1991, Oxford University.

Stringer M, Pablot SM, Brereton R: Paediatric intussusception, *Br J Surg* 79(9):867, 1992.

Tanagho E, McAninch J: *Smith's general urology,* ed 13, Norwalk, Conn, 1992, Appleton & Lange.

Van-Why S et al: Abdominal symptoms as presentation of hypertensive crisis, *Am J Dis Child* 147(6):638, 1993.

Yamada T et al: *Textbook of gastroenterology,* 2 vols, 1991, Lippincott.

RECOMMENDED READING

Spiro H: An internist's approach to acute abdominal pain, *Med Clin North Am* 77(5):963, 1993.

9 | Musculoskeletal Problems

Functioning of the musculoskeletal system is paramount for mobility. Complaints involving this system warrant careful evaluation and communication with the patient in order to allay unnecessary fears and to convey information regarding the assessment process and potential outcomes. Understanding the normal anatomy and physiology of the musculoskeletal system is necessary for an accurate assessment of injuries and illness involving this system. It is also important to realize that systemic illnesses may become evident as symptoms in the musculoskeletal system. A broad knowledge base of medical problems is helpful in the accurate assessment of the severity and nature of patient complaints involving the musculoskeletal system.

When patients have injuries or illnesses affecting the musculoskeletal system, the goal of health care providers is to maintain "life and limb." Naturally, this is usually the goal of patients as well, and in their pain and fear it is helpful for them to know that their health care providers will work to provide them with pain relief and treatment that are necessary for restoring optimal musculoskeletal function.

TRIAGE HISTORY

Taking a history in triage of a patient with a complaint involving the musculoskeletal system typically involves an on-the-spot determination of whether the complaint is injury related. If the complaint is injury related, the triage professional makes a brief determination immediately on the severity of the injury and the necessity for first aid or a more thorough triage evaluation. During the triage history the nurse takes into account the patient's age and developmental status, since these are important in understanding the likely implications of injuries. For example, in all ankle injuries of young children avulsion fractures are much more likely than ligamentous injury, so immobilization and x-ray of the affected area are crucial to appropriate diagnosis (Harkless and Krych, 1990).

In any patient with escalating or persistent edema it is almost always helpful to elevate the patient's affected extremity and apply ice if the edema is injury related (see discussion of ischemic myositis in Deformity section). If the patient's presenting complaint is obviously severe, for example, an open fracture, the affected limb is immobilized and treated with the appropriate temporary dressings and the patient enters the triage area for a brief but concise history before emergent triage into the emergency department (ED). When a musculoskeletal complaint is not injury related, the nurse must determine the time and manner of symptom onset and get a concise understanding of the relationship between symptoms and time factors. Severity of symptoms should be determined using functional indicators relative to the patient's activities of daily living and job-related activities. If symptoms are work related, triage may involve entering the patient into a system that deals with worker's compensation. It is important that the interviewer question the patient about repetitive work or sports demands on the hands, fingers, or other extremities relevant to the chief complaint.

When it is apparent that musculoskeletal symptoms are secondary to systemic problems, questions pertinent to assessing relevant systems should be incorporated into the triage interview. When a patient has musculoskeletal symptoms that are related to an injury, specific questions regarding the nature of the injury and physics of the affected body part(s) should be asked. For example, patients entering triage with a complaint of ankle pain that was precipitated by a fall while playing basketball should be asked whether they fell while jumping or running, how they fell (e.g., forward or backward), the position of the ankle at the time of the fall, whether any unusual sounds were heard (e.g., a pop, snap, or crack), and whether they continued to play or immediately rested. Although it may seem that the triage nurse is searching for minutiae, determination of the sequence of the injury is helpful in determining the severity and extent of injury. For example, an injury to the medial ankle is much more severe and indicates a greater likelihood that invasive treatment may be necessary, and patients with this type of injury should be triaged with a higher acuity level (Harkless and Krych, 1990). Treatment

| BOX 9-1 | History Questions for Patients With Musculoskeletal Complaints |

- When did the problem begin?
- What did you notice at the time of the injury (pain, deformity)?
- Describe the injury that led to your symptoms; specifically, did you hear any popping, cracking, snapping, or other obvious sounds at the time of the injury?
- How did you land when you fell (or "came off the bicycle" or the like)?
- Besides the symptom you came here to have evaluated, have you noticed any other symptoms?
- Describe your discomfort. Specifically, on a scale of 1 to 10, with 10 being the worst pain you've ever felt, how bad is your pain or discomfort right now?
- Did you walk (or use the affected extremity or joint) after the injury?
- Have your symptoms been continuous or intermittent?

at the time of the injury should also be determined. Important history questions to ask a patient with a chief complaint related to the musculoskeletal system are summarized in Box 9–1.

When parents or caretakers of pediatric patients complain that a child has frequent injuries or describe the child as "clumsy," the triage nurse should be alert to the possibility that the child may have problems with vision, a rotational deformity, neurologic problems, or muscle disease (Ehrlich et al., 1992). The triage nurse should take a moment to ask about the pattern of the frequent injuries and the manifestation of the child's coordination problems.

When an injury is suspected to be related to abuse or violence, communication with the appropriate agency personnel (e.g., child protective services, licensing, or law enforcement) is necessary. Triage professionals must use intuition regarding the degree to which the interview should be conducted. If they deem that the patient may not stay for evaluation or treatment or if the triage professional is placed at risk through contact with potentially violent significant others, questions regarding abuse are best deferred until the patient is in the ED.

PHYSICAL ASSESSMENT

Physical assessment of the musculoskeletal system should be consistent, whether the patient's symptoms are related to medical problems or an injury. After the patient's vital signs have been obtained, assessment of the range of motion (ROM) of the affected and opposite extremity should be performed. Although a thorough approach to assessing ROM should include, in order, active, passive, and resistive ROM, it may be practical to assess only active ROM (the nurse asks the patient to demonstrate the ability to move the joint in every normal position to the fullest extent comfortable). It is important that the patient demonstrate mobility proficiency (active ROM) rather than the nurse assessing passive ROM (the patient is asked to relax and the nurse moves the limb for the patient) so that inadvertent injury or pain induced by the professional's manipulation of the extremity, should the nurse take the patient beyond a point of limitation during passive ROM, is prevented. If there is limitation during

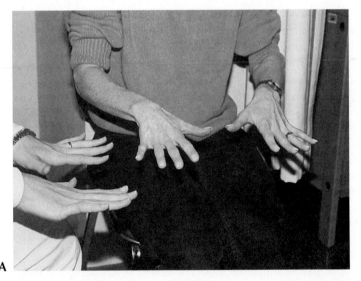

A

Fig. 9–1   A, Active range of motion should always be assessed first to determine the patient's abilities to perform ROMs. The examiner may model the movements to be performed if the patient finds it helpful.

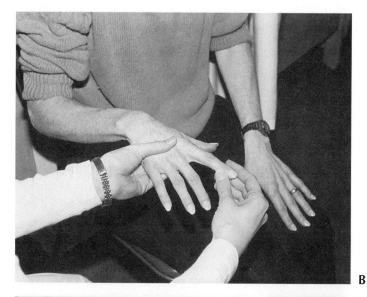

B

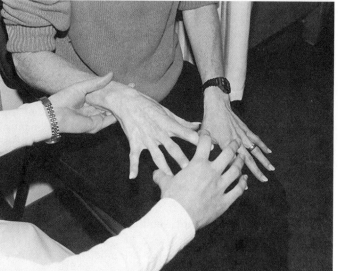

C

Fig. 9–1, cont'd   B, During passive ROM, the examiner assesses for crepitation, popping, and muscle tone abnormalities. **C,** Resistive ROM exercises enable the examiner to assess patient strength against resistance.

active ROM, the nurse should record which ROM is limited and the reason, for example, "patient unable to abduct at the shoulder >90 degrees during active ROM due to severe pain." If the patient's chief complaint is weakness and the patient is unable to perform active ROM, the degree to which the patient is mobile should be recorded, and passive ROM should be determined during the personnel's assessment of the patient. Resistive ROM is also performed during a more thorough assessment of the patient's musculoskeletal system unless contraindicated, although for certain neurologic complaints assessing resistive ROM is highly appropriate during triage. Symmetry of ROM and strength should always be evaluated, taking into consideration that the patient's dominant side is typically stronger than the nondominant side (Fig. 9–1).

Vital assessments that should be performed on all patients with musculoskeletal complaints include evaluation of extremity color, temperature, sensation, and pulses and comparison of the affected extremity with the opposing extremity for symmetry. Considering the patient's overall pigmentation, the lighting in the triage area, and comparison with all extremities is important when assessing pigmentation. Dark-skinned patients may be asked whether they have noticed a change in the color of the affected extremity, and their response recorded along with the triage nurse's observations. This information is helpful in all patients but may be more valuable when light-skinned nurses question their own impressions because of lack of experience or uncertainty in evaluating the integument of persons of color. Temperature of a patient's extremity should be assessed with the dorsal side of the examiner's hand, which is more sensitive to temperature. The extremities should be evaluated bilaterally and distally to proximally, again with consideration to the patient's overall emotional and physical condition (Fig. 9–2). Sensation should be assessed during the history by asking whether the patient has numbness, anesthesia, or paresthesia in any extremity or extremity part. During the physical assessment portion of the triage assessment, sensation may be grossly determined by having the patient close his/her eyes and touching the patient with a tongue blade or another blunt object, asking the patient to identify when the touch occurs. Peripheral pulses that should be examined include

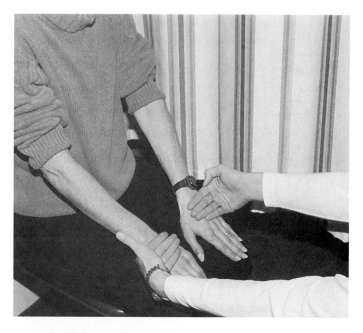

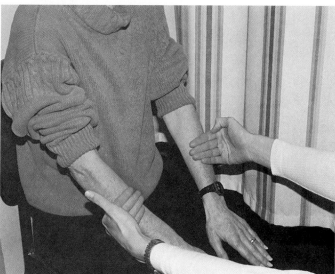

Fig. 9–2 Temperature evaluation of extremities proceeds distal to proximal.

| BOX 9–2 | **Physical Assessment of the Musculoskeletal System in Triage** |

- Evaluate peripheral pulses distal and proximal to the site of pain.
- Evaluate for joint deformity.
- Evaluate location, radiation, severity of discomfort.
- Evaluate extremity or affected part distally to proximally and compare for symmetric color.
- Examiner uses the dorsum of her/his hand to evaluate temperature of affected part, noting anatomic demarcations for asymmetric temperature changes or excessive coolness or warmth.
- Examiner evaluates range of motion (active, passive, and resistive) thoroughly in all possible ranges of affected extremity and compares with opposite extremity for symmetry.
- Examiner evaluates sensation symmetrically and distally to proximally, using cotton wisp and safety pin or unfolded paper clip.

pulses both distal and proximal to an injured area when an injury is present. The evaluation of the presence and symmetry of pulses is sufficient in the triage setting. Physical assessment techniques to be performed in triage on the patient with a complaint involving the musculoskeletal system are summarized in Box 9–2.

Physical assessment findings are recorded in the triage record using bony landmarks, major muscle groups, and anatomic terminology as references for describing the location of normal, positive, or negative physical examination findings. Recording assessment findings on an ''anatomic'' figure is also a concise way of indicating the location of abnormal findings such as ecchymoses, lacerations, and deformities.

The physical assessment is guided by the patient's history with particular attention to areas most likely to be affected by reported discomfort. Critical history and physical information gleaned in triage that cues the examiner that the adult or pediatric patient should be immediately seen in the ED for care is summarized in Boxes 9–3 and 9–4. The triage nurse should not

BOX 9-3	Critical Findings That Cue Emergent Triage Designation for Care in Emergency Department

- Diminished or absent pulses with or without clinical history indicative of arterial damage (may confirm absent pulses with Doppler instrument in triage if available)
- Asymmetric pallor or cyanosis of any extremity or extremity part
- Extreme temperature abnormalities (e.g., coolness or warmth) with clinical history significant for vascular injury, infection, or fracture
- Open fracture
- Anesthesia at site of injury or distal or proximal to site of injury
- Presentation or history consistent with emergent musculoskeletal problems such as compartment syndrome, aneurysm, arterial injury, or acute arterial insufficiency
- Potential for spinal cord injury

BOX 9-4	Pediatric Alert: Cues for Emergent Triage Designation for Care in Emergency Department

- Weakness and lethargy
- Fractured femur (trauma)
- Weight loss
- Presentation consistent with suspected child abuse

be reticent to triage the patient as emergent when even one indicator that life or limb is threatened is evident during the patient's evaluation.

WEAKNESS

Patients who complain of generalized weakness may have primary musculoskeletal problems, but their symptoms may be caused by systemic problems such as fluid and electrolyte imbalance, infection, or neuromuscular problems such as multiple sclerosis or by medication, street drug, or alcohol ingestion. Assessment of the patient with generalized weakness should include history questions that ferret out the suddenness or chronicity of the symptom onset and the degree to which the patient is impaired by weakness. The patient should be asked about the degree of impairment resulting from weakness by using functional ranges of home and work activities. Specific questions in the triage history may include questions regarding medications, infectious diseases (e.g., trichinosis), and exposure to pesticides or other chemicals. Review of questions relevant to possible systemic problems should be considered, as appropriate, in relation to anemia, cardiopulmonary disease, chronic inflammatory disease, chronic infections such as human immunodefi-

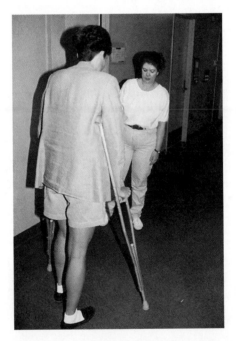

Fig. 9–3 Gait assessment in triage provides understanding regarding appropriate technique used with assistive devices and limitations related to pain or weakness.

ciency virus (HIV), malignancy, depression, and fibromyalgia. Malingering and deconditioning should also be considered during the history and triage designation (Kelley et al., 1993).

Physical assessment of patients with weakness should include observation of the patient's gait; observed difficulty or discomfort with ambulation and the distance that the patient was observed ambulating should be recorded. These observations are helpful references during the reevaluation period, when the patient's disposition and risk for falls or complications are being determined. The patient's use of walking aids such as canes or a walker should also be recorded during the triage assessment (Fig. 9–3). If weakness is reported to be limb specific, active ROM should be evaluated. In patients with weakness, passive ROM is typically greater than active ROM, since the patient's limitation of movement is not due to pain or joint mobility difficulties but rather to muscle weakness. If the triage nurse evaluates passive ROM, care should still be taken not to perform the assessment too rapidly, since it is conceivable that contractures may have begun in the patient with chronic and progressive weakness who is not responsive to or receiving the beneficial effects of physical therapy (Fig. 9–4). Muscle tone can briefly be evaluated by bilateral palpation of exposed mus-

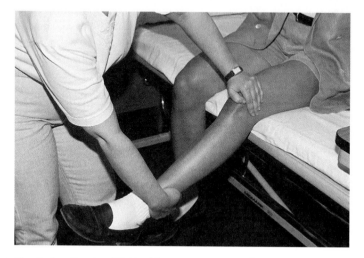

Fig. 9–4   Passive ROM of lower extremities (knee extension).

BOX 9–5	**Key Points* in Triage Record for Patients With Weakness**

- Is the patient's weakness objectively apparent or strictly subjective?
- Is the patient's weakness generalized or localized?
- Is the patient's weakness asymmetric or symmetric?
- Is there a specific pattern or is the weakness distal or proximal?

From Kelley et al., eds: *Textbook of rheumatology,* ed 4, Philadelphia, 1993, WB Saunders.
*In addition to the usual triage history questions and vital signs.

cles, and their atrophy or hypertonicity recorded. Furthermore, if obvious spasticity, flaccidity, or fasciculations are discovered in any muscle groups during assessment of passive ROM, this finding should be recorded. The patient's weakness should be summarized in the triage note (Box 9–5).

When weakness is reported to be a problem in children, the triage nurse should be astute in observing for signs of systemic problems such as dehydration or diabetes. Children who have weakness and are unable to perform the work of play are often gravely ill or are suffering from failure to thrive, and the triage professional must triage these patients not only according to their vital signs but also according to general appearance and risk of problems relevant to the chief complaint. Pediatric patients with weakness should also be asked about appetite, nutrition, and weight loss (Fig. 9–5). A scale weight must be obtained, and a record of the patient's most recent scale weight as reported by the care provider also recorded. Immediate triage for ED care should occur in pediatric patients with weakness accompanied by lethargy and an inability to stand and walk (when age appropriate).

PAIN

Before evaluating the possible origins and severity of a problem causing patients to feel pain the triage nurse should consider the patient's psychologic state and level of fatigue, since these

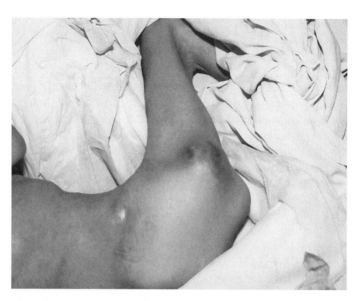

Fig. 9–5 Emaciation and contractures in a pediatric patient.

factors greatly influence the patient's perception of pain (Harkless and Krych, 1990). Patients with anxiety and exhaustion should be made as comfortable as possible; recognition of their state of being may help them relax and develop a relationship of trust with the triage nurse, an excellent foundation for trusting and participating in care once they are seen in the ED.

Musculoskeletal pain may be present as a result of trauma or inflammation of muscles, joints, or supporting ligaments and tendons. It must be determined whether the patient can identify precipitating events or factors that are relevant to the pain. As the triage nurse considers the location of the patient's pain, closed-ended questions should be asked regarding changes in equipment or clothing affecting the musculoskeletal system (e.g., shoes), when the change occurred, changes in the surface or location of activities, and specific changes in activity. Personal changes that may also be precipitating factors in musculoskeletal pain include a new job with new activities involving the musculoskeletal system, a change in job role, a change in family life, or a change in living situation that may require more walking, stair climbing, or carrying of items such as groceries for greater distances (Harkless and Krych, 1990). Whether the pain is continuous, intermittent, or present at rest or only during activities that aggravate discomfort should also be determined. The triage nurse must pay careful attention to information regarding the manner of onset of pain and precipitating factors. Patients who have fallen or have had traumatic injuries more than 24 hours before arrival at triage should not be assumed to have only inflammation. Fractures, whether traumatic or pathologic, may cause increasingly severe, continuous pain as time progresses, even though the initial discomfort may not have been noticeable or severe. It is crucial for all triage nurses to be familiar with the cardinal signs of fracture (Box 9–6) and also to realize that not all patients with a fracture have the cardinal signs (Adams and Hamblen, 1992).

Evaluation of subjective pain must include a description of the pain. If the patient is unable to volunteer adjectives for describing pain, it may be necessary to give examples of descriptions, to ascertain the type of pain the patient feels.

Determining the type of pain is helpful in distinguishing the possible severity of the problem and, subsequently, the appropriate triage level designation. Specific location and radiation of the pain are determined by asking the patient to specifically indicate the area of discomfort, beginning with the area with the worst pain, and severity should be evaluated using the severity scale (from 1 to 10). Inquiry into the use of palliative factors should include questions regarding the use of hot

---

| BOX 9–6 | **Triage Cues to the Presence of a Fracture** |

- Obvious or palpable deformity
- Edema localized to injured area
- Ecchymosis
- Point tenderness over fracture
- Impaired function
- Abnormal mobility (joint moves in abnormal direction)
- Crepitation or grating

BOX 9–7	**Problems Commonly Associated With Musculoskeletal Pain and Triage Cues**

CARPAL TUNNEL SYNDROME

Numbness and tingling that awakens the patient in the night or early morning; Phalen's sign; Tinel's sign

CELLULITIS

Constant, unrelenting, burning pain; edema; localized erythema or red streaks from affected area; warm to touch

CONSTANT NERVE PRESSURE (SUCH AS EDEMA, MASS)

Constant, unrelenting, burning pain

LOCAL NERVE IMPINGEMENT, INDUCED BY TIGHT CLOTHING OR CHRONIC PROCESS

Burning pain aggravated by activity but relieved by rest

DIABETIC NEUROPATHY

Burning, superficial pain, often with paresthesias, may interfere with ability to fall asleep

OCCLUSIVE ARTERIAL DISEASE

Sharp, stabbing, deep, aching pain that may awaken patient or be induced by activity; may awaken a sleeping patient; rarely relieved by pain medication, but may be relieved by dependent position of limb

ISCHEMIC LIMB

Cold extremity, atrophic skin, absent hair growth, dystrophic nails, delayed capillary refill, intermittent claudication

FRACTURE

Obvious or palpable deformity; edema localized to injured or painful area; ecchymosis; point tenderness over fracture; impaired function; abnormal mobility; crepitation or grating; high-risk patient profile (such as osteoporosis, overuse, cancer)

OVERUSE INJURIES (SPORTS OR WORK RELATED)

Hisk-risk history; edema and pain; identifiable precipitating factors

Continued.

BOX 9–7	Problems Commonly Associated With Musculoskeletal Pain and Triage Cues— cont'd

CHRONIC ORTHOPEDIC OR NEUROMUSCULAR SYNDROMES SUCH AS MULTIPLE SCLEROSIS, RHEUMATOID ARTHRITIS

Weakness; disuse atrophy; symptoms specific to disease process

SPINAL CORD COMPRESSION

Back pain or radicular pain that is dull, aching, constant, and aggravated by lying down, coughing, sneezing, passing stool, activity; may be unilateral or bilateral; leg weakness may be present

SPRAIN, TEARS, MUSCLE RUPTURE, STRAINS, OR ACUTE INFLAMMATION OF TENDON OR LIGAMENTOUS SUPPORTING STRUCTURES

Common in court sports, sprints, baseball, softball, sports played on uneven terrain; severe pain in muscle strains and ruptures commonly involving gastrocnemius-soleus complex, posterior tibial muscle, and peroneal muscles; seen in individuals with poor warm-up and training or overuse of muscles in a pronated or flat-footed individual, particularly if the patient is overweight and does not wear supportive shoes

---

or cold compresses or treatments, topical ointments or medications (e.g., Ben-Gay), oral medications (nonprescription, prescribed for the patient, or prescribed for and borrowed from another), and home remedies. It is helpful for nurses to be familiar with terminology common to the individual regarding home remedies used for musculoskeletal pain, such as liniments and mustard or pepper plasters. If the nurse is unfamiliar with home remedies that a patient may be using, a simple descriptor of the method and contents and effectiveness of the remedy is sufficient.

Because pain is a distressing symptom, the triage nurse should be alert to ways in which the patient's pain can be minimized during a necessary waiting period. Pain involving an extremity may cue the examiner that the extremity or affected part should be immobilized and elevated to minimize associated edema and that a compression dressing should be applied, if indicated. Furthermore, patients with intolerable pain (from the patient's point of view) should be triaged as emergent, since unrelieved pain causes the release of catecholamines which, in turn, increases inflammation and eventually results in delay of the healing process. The use of a calm voice and manner by the triage nurse, coupled with education regarding the treatment and triage process and relaxed breathing, can also have a calming effect on many patients, which may result in diminished perception of pain.

The triage professional should have a strong knowledge base in diagnoses associated with various common pain presentations. This knowledge base leads to triage assessments that are appropriate for the patient's symptoms and appropriate triage. Common musculoskeletal problems and associated triage cues are presented in Box 9–7.

CERVICAL INJURIES AND SPINAL CORD PROBLEMS

Pain involving structures in the neck or spine may trigger an intuitive sense that use of a cervical spine collar is indicated. Indications for cervical spine collars should be clear in the mind of the triage professional, however, so that intuition is not the only tool the nurse relies on, particularly since patients can have a spinal cord injury without neck or back pain (Box 9–8). Indications for cervical spine precautions include head injury, falls involving loss of consciousness, and falls or injuries with tenderness or pain at the neck or cervical spine point. Fractures involving the cervical spine or atlas that are not suspected early

---

| **BOX 9–8** | **Indications for Cervical Spine Precautions** |

- History of trauma to head, neck, or back with or without resultant neck or back pain (''whiplash,'' hanging, falls, penetrating trauma, blunt force trauma)
- History of neck pain associated with traumatic injury
- Sensory or motor deficits (tingling, numbness, weakness, paralysis)
- Spinal deformity

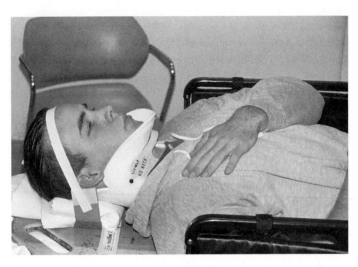

Fig. 9–6 C-spine precautions should be taken immediately for any patient at risk for spinal cord injury.

and met with swift intervention may result in paralysis or death (Fig. 9–6).

The areas of the spine at greatest risk for damage resulting from injury are the cervical and lumbar regions. Patients with complaints of pain in these areas or with radiating back pain after traumatic injury should be treated with caution. Infrequently, patients may arrive at triage with a history of traumatic injury for which they were evaluated and cleared, but they return to the ED days or weeks after the initial injury because of neurologic deficits. These patients may have spinal cord injury without radiographic abnormality (SCIWORA), a syndrome. These patients have no visible bony damage to the spinal column on x-ray, but damage has occurred to the spinal cord. This syndrome more frequently occurs in children because of the elasticity of their spinal connective tissue. All patients with a history of head, neck, or back trauma who are considered to be at high risk for this syndrome should be given a cervical collar and treated with great caution (Laskowski-Jones, 1993).

Spinal cord damage occurs not only in patients with traumatic injury but also in patients with metastatic cancers that spread to the spine and cause compression of the cord or weakness of the vertebra (Peterson, 1993). Compression of the spine is most common with cancers of the prostate, breast, and lung, so patients with a history of these cancers who complain of back pain, even if associating the discomfort with activity, should have the possibility of compression considered, and they should be triaged as emergent. Weakness of the legs is another common symptom of spinal compression, as is radicular pain (radiating on the dermatome of the affected vertebra's spinal nerve root). The concert of sudden, severe pain followed by weakness must be recognized as a potentially critical condition, and these patients should be triaged for immediate care (*American Journal of Nursing,* 1993).

Patients with back pain should be carefully queried about precipitating factors to the pain. Sports that involve twisting actions may precipitate muscle, ligament, or spine injuries, and the triage nurse should include closed-ended questions regarding sports and dance activities in interviewing patients with musculoskeletal pain.

UPPER EXTREMITY PAIN

It is helpful, when evaluating upper extremity discomfort, to have the patient specify the exact area of discomfort and evaluate the time pattern of pain. Associated symptoms can also be key to appropriate diagnosis. For example, the patient with carpal tunnel syndrome typically complains of numbness and tingling that awakens the patient during the night or in the early morning hours with burning pain and loss of light touch in the thumb and first two fingers. The results of Phalen's test and Tinel's sign will be positive; if the triage nurse has time to perform these procedures, the results may be of interest (Cailliet, 1991).

Understanding precipitating factors to upper extremity pain is key to appropriate triage designation and assessment. Knowing the forces involved in recreational and athletic activities the patient participates in helps the triage nurse anticipate the type of injury the patient has had. In the athlete who throws a ball overhand, the shoulder is vulnerable to injury because repetitive, high-energy forces are involved and the activity is prolonged (Kvitne and Jobe, 1993). Unless there is extreme discomfort or circulatory compromise the patient can safely be triaged as urgent in most instances. Many athletes who are injured are immediately concerned about the implications of their injuries to their livelihood or sport involvement. Although the triage nurse cannot diagnose the problem she/he can educate the patient during treatment of the extremity about the importance of immediate rest, use of ice, and elevation of the extremity, if appropriate, and use of appropriate equipment and considerations of timing when they receive a medical release to perform again. The ulnar nerve is vulnerable to injury at the wrist in activities that cause repetitive trauma or compression to the wrist, such as bicycling, weight lifting, gymnastics, and martial arts (Hainline, 1994). The patient should be encouraged to change hand position during exercises such as bicycling, and she/he should be encouraged to use supportive equipment if necessary in sports such as weight lifting. Patient education in triage regarding injury prevention is practical only if time permits.

LOWER EXTREMITY PAIN

Pain in the lower extremities may occur in patients with medical problems and may be significant but not critical, or pain in the lower extremities may occur as a result of trauma or injuries caused by overuse.

Medical patients with diabetes and those with a history of circulation problems are at high risk for critical problems of the lower extremities. The triage nurse must be aware of the signs and symptoms of arterial occlusion, since this problem necessitates emergent triage into the ED for care (Box 9–8).

Injuries associated with overuse, such as stress fractures of the ankles and feet, are common in athletes and in patients with menstrual irregularity, osteoporosis, diabetes or idiopathic neuropathy, smoking and alcohol intake, hypothyroidism, anorexia nervosa, Paget's disease, and rheumatoid arthritis (Eisele and Sammarco, 1993). Fatigue or stress fractures may develop as a result of excessive stress placed on normal bones or the failure of abnormal bone to function in the presence of normal demands. Presenting signs and symptoms of stress or fatigue fractures include edema and point tenderness at the site of the stress fracture; the patient may have a history of previous stress fractures.

The sex of the patient is significant in considering possible problems. In many children, particularly girls, dislocation of the patella is common and causes swelling and pain medial to the patella; the patella sometimes relocates spontaneously and without obvious cause (e.g., on rising from a chair) (Ehrlich et al., 1992). The triage nurse should carefully examine the knee if it is relevant to the patient's chief complaint.

Older children commonly arrive at triage because of an earlier injury involving the lower extremities when they have not allowed the injured area to heal adequately. The triage nurse should ask the patient about treatment, follow-up, and current activities when they report discomfort associated with an earlier injury.

DEFORMITY AND FRACTURES

Patients with a chief complaint of deformity arrive at triage either with an acute injury or with a problem related to a chronic, debilitating condition. Acute-onset deformity is most frequently seen in association with fractures and may be highly distressing to the patient. When fractures with deformity occur, it is important to immobilize the extremity by the application of a temporary splint or, in the case of a hip fracture, by immobilizing the patient. Although deformity alerts a nurse that a fracture is likely, the triage nurse must be aware that not all fractures cause deformity; in fact, triage may be difficult in the case of vague or minimal symptoms. For that reason, the triage nurse should be alert to the risk factors for nontraumatic fractures such as insufficiency stress fractures, which are common in frail, elderly white women with a history of osteoporosis (Tountas, 1993). Risk factors for the "worst case" possibilities must be considered when designating the patient's triage level, since delay in treatment increases the risk of morbidity and mortality.

The area of trauma should be examined closely for open fracture sites. When an open fracture exists, a light, sterile, non-stick dressing should be applied over the area. Any clothing restricting blood flow should be cut to allow free circulation. Assessment of proximal and distal pulses should be performed and documented, even in the absence of "pumping" blood flow from the area of the open fracture. Any patient with an open fracture should be triaged as emergent for ED care, since an

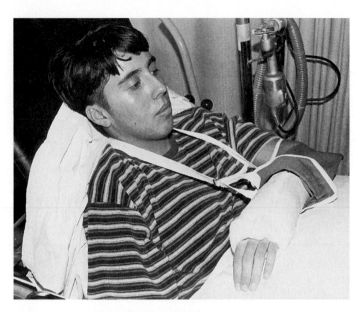

Fig. 9–7   The cast is split to decrease the risk of edema and impaired circulation, which are common in the first 24 to 48 hours after traumatic injury.

increased risk of morbidity is associated with infection and circulation problems when treatment is delayed (Fig. 9–7). The remainder of the neurovascular assessment may be performed in the ED, since early treatment is crucial.

Patients with deformity concurrent with a closed fracture should have the extremity immobilized with a splint and be triaged to the radiography department or into the ED as soon as possible, particularly when the patient has severe pain. Neurovascular checks should be performed immediately and at intervals when departmental treatment is delayed. The triage nurse may order an extremity x-ray, if that is consistent with hospital policy. The triage nurse may educate the patient that not all fractures can be diagnosed immediately on x-ray and that follow-up care after ED evaluation is always helpful, even if fracture is not present or diagnosed and soft tissue injuries are the cause of pain or abnormal limb appearance. Stress fractures,

BOX 9–9	**Signs and Symptoms of Compartment Syndrome (Ischemic Myositis)**

- Progressive edema
- Pain exceeding that expected for the injury received
- Severe, increasing pain with passive range of motion
- Sensory deficit (early finding)
- Weakness that may progress to paralysis
- Pulselessness (late finding)

for example, most common in the lesser metatarsals of the fore-foot, cannot be diagnosed immediately on x-ray; in fact, they are not usually visualized on radiographs until 2 to 3 weeks after the injury. The nurse may suspect this problem if the patient complains of calcaneal pain and reports activities at high risk for this problem, such as aerobics and running (activities performed primarily on the ball of the foot) (Harkless and Krych, 1990).

Triage professionals must be particularly alert to the potential for ischemic myositis (compartment syndrome), which may occur when there is an acute, critical interruption in blood flow to muscles (Box 9–9). The many precipitants of this problem include arthroscopy, infusion of intravenous fluids, injury, burns, and prolonged tourniquet use (Gold et al., 1993; Rodeo et al., 1993; Sheridan et al., 1994; Sneyd et al., 1993). Elevation and ice, commonly used in early treatment of fractures and sprains, increase the patient's perception of pain in the presence of compartment syndrome, since these therapeutic measures reduce blood flow even more dramatically (Fig. 9–8). Without early detection and immediate medical treatment ischemic myositis can lead to permanent loss of limb function and systemic complications such as renal failure (Swearingen, 1990).

One common cause of deformity in pediatric patients is "nursemaid's elbow," or elbow dislocation that results from a child being quickly jerked or pulled by one arm. Typically the child does not perform an active range of motion or reach—which the examiner can assess by offering the child a bright object, toy, or puppet on the affected side—as is evident in the

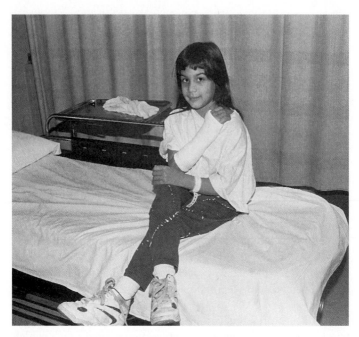

Fig. 9–8   Edema is minimized by instructing the patient to hold the injured arm above the level of the heart.

child's inability to move the affected side. Unless there is neurovascular impairment, this condition, although distressing to the care provider and child, is not designated as emergent.

Child abuse is a possible cause of fracture. Whenever possible, the verbally capable child should be questioned about the cause of the injury before the triage nurse questions the accompanying adult. Cues in triage that child abuse may be involved (Box 9–10) include delay in seeking treatment and the age of the patient. In infants under 1 year of age accidental fractures are extremely rare, and they are uncommon in children under 3 years of age (Carty, 1993). It is important for the triage nurse to observe and document indications of child abuse and to activate child protective services or to communicate that need in the nursing orders so that the child's safety can be addressed

BOX 9–10	**Triage Cues for Potential Child Abuse**

- Delay in seeking treatment
- Apparent fracture in a child under 3 years of age*
- Rib fractures, scapular fractures, fractures of the outer end of the clavicle
- Finger injuries in children not yet walking
- Head injury
- Child in the care of another child
- Caretaker ignorance or carelessness, gleaned during triage history*
- Historian's focus on the child's behavior
- Change in events of the history
- Injury more severe than is reasonable for the reported history†

*From Kowal-Vern A et al: *Clin Pediatr* 11:653, 1992.
†From Leventhal J et al: *Am J Dis Child* 147(1):87, 1993.

BOX 9–11	**Triage Treatment of Patients With a Musculoskeletal Problem**

- Provide a wheelchair or gurney if necessary for safety or comfort whenever possible, or assist patient into position of comfort.
- Apply dressing to wounds as needed.
- Rest, elevate, and ice the injury, and use a compression dressing if indicated.
- Immobilize deformed joint or extremity that is a source of severe pain.
- Educate patient about when to inform triage nurse of changes in signs or symptoms during the waiting period.
- If surgery is likely or if the patient is nauseated because of severe discomfort, place patient on a regimen of receiving nothing by mouth.
- Provide emesis basin and cool washcloth if needed.
- Provide age-appropriate toy or stickers for pediatric patient if available.

immediately. Children with a high index of suspicion should be triaged into the ED immediately, since delay in treatment may cause the parent or person accompanying the child to leave the ED before the child receives care. Child abuse is the leading cause of death in 6- to 12-month-old infants and the second leading cause of death in infants 1 to 6 months of age (Cooper, 1992). The triage nurse must always err on the side of vigilance in the case of injured children. Similar concerns exist in responding to the potential reality of domestic violence. The system for dealing with domestic violence should be activated from the point of triage if necessary. All possible perpetrators of violence against patients being seen in the ED should be kept from entering the ED, and security services should be notified for the safety of the patient and the triage nurse.

Patients who enter the ED with chief complaints involving the musculoskeletal system need careful evaluation and comfort measures, which decrease their anxiety and discomfort. Depending on the problem, the triage nurse should initiate comfort measures in the triage area whenever possible. Triage treatment options for the patient with a musculoskeletal problem are summarized in Box 9–11.

REFERENCES

Adams J, Hamblen D: *Outline of fractures,* ed 10, New York, 1992, Churchill Livingstone.

Cailliet R: *Neck and arm pain,* Philadelphia, 1991, FA Davis.

Carty H: Fractures caused by child abuse, *J Bone Joint Surg (Br)* 75(6):849, 1993.

Cooper A: Thoracoabdominal trauma. In Ludwig S, Kornberg A, eds: *Child abuse: a medical reference,* New York, 1992, Churchill Livingstone.

Critical difference: spinal cord compression, *Am J Nurs* 93(1):56, 1993.

Ehrlich M, Hulstyn M, d'Amato C: Sports injuries in children and the clumsy child, *Pediatr Clin North Am* 39(3):433, 1992.

Eisele S, Sammarco G: Fatigue fractures of the foot and ankle in the athlete, *J Bone Joint Surg (Am)* 75(2):290, 1993.

Gold M, Bleday R, Brown F: Complications of prolonged bilateral lower extremity tourniquet, *Plast Reconstr Surg* 91(1):198, 1993.

Hainline B: Nerve injuries, *Med Clin North Am* 78(2):327, 1994.

Harkless L, Krych S: *Handbook of common foot problems,* New York, 1990, Churchill Livingstone.

Kelley W et al, eds: *Textbook of rheumatology,* ed 4, Philadelphia, 1993, WB Saunders.

Kowal-Vern A et al: Fractures in the under-3-year-old age cohort, *Clin Pediatr* 31(11):653, 1992.

Kvitne R, Jobe F: The diagnosis and treatment of anterior instability in the throwing athlete, *Clin Orthop* 291:107, 1993.

Laskowski-Jones L: Acute SCI: how to minimize the damage, *Am J Nurs* 93(12):22, 1993.

Leventhal J et al: Fractures in young children: distinguishing child abuse from unintentional injuries, *Am J Dis Child* 147(1):87, 1993.

Peterson R: A nursing intervention for early detection of spinal cord compressions in patients with cancer, *Cancer Nurs* 16(2):113, 1993.

Rodeo S, Forster R, Wiland A: Neurological complications due to arthroscopy, *J Bone Joint Surg (Am)* 75(6):917, 1993.

Sheridan R, Tompkins R, McManus W: Intracompartment sepsis in burn patients, *J Trauma* 36(3):301, 1994.

Sneyd J, Lau W, McLaren I: Forearm compartment syndrome following intravenous infusion with a manual ''bulb'' pump, *Anesth Analg* 76(5):1160, 1993.

Swearingen P: *Manual of nursing therapeutics: applying nursing diagnoses to medical disorders,* ed 2, St. Louis, 1990, Mosby.

Tountas A: Insufficiency stress fractures of the femoral neck in elderly women, *Clin Orthop* 292:202, 1993.

RECOMMENDED READING

Aloia J: *A colour atlas of osteoporosis,* St Louis, 1993, Mosby.

10 Integument Problems

Patient complaints related to the integument may be indicative of disease in the integument, or they may signify systemic problems originating in other organs. The triage nurse must have a strong knowledge base of many systemic diseases, as well as familiarity with common skin disorders, to correctly triage patients with integument abnormalities. In addition to a strong knowledge base, the triage nurse must have excellent interviewing skills and the ability to rapidly perform a physical assessment of the patient's integument. The two most important questions a triage nurse typically thinks of when evaluating a patient with integument problems are the following: Does the patient have a contagious infection? Is the skin problem indicative of a critical or life-threatening problem? If the triage nurse is busy with a number of difficult patients and a patient with an integument problem arrives at triage, the triage nurse must make a rapid determination about whether the patient can wait in the waiting area with other patients or must wait in an isolated waiting area. The second decision the triage nurse must make is whether the patient needs to be evaluated as quickly as possible or can wait. Again, the only way that the triage nurse is prepared to make these crucial decisions is by having a clear knowledge base of common infectious diseases and life-threatening disorders with signs and symptoms involving the integument.

Determination of triage acuity for problems in the integument and subsequent diagnosis and treatment will eventually be made more scientific through the use of computerized databases that cue the professional to consider various possibilities based on signs and symptoms of the patient. Ultimately the triage professional and emergency department (ED) care providers must make an assessment, but references that are available to help detect critical problems associated with integument or any other systemic signs and symptoms should be considered useful and may be lifesaving (Simon, 1992).

The triage nurse must be wary of patients with problems in the integument who want a quick decision about whether they need to be seen in the ED or can wait and be seen by their primary care provider at a later time. Even pediatric patients who arrive at triage for identification of chicken pox (varicella) should be categorized as urgent and seen in the ED, since life-threatening complications of this common childhood virus do occur, such as group A beta-hemolytic streptococcal infections (GABHS), and a cursory look at a patient and subsequent dismissal would be dangerous and not helpful (Cowan et al., 1994) (Fig. 10–1). There are odd occasions when patients have simple problems involving the integument, such as having the fingers stuck together with superglue. If ED policy permits and the triage nurse can assist the patient in ungluing the fingers by

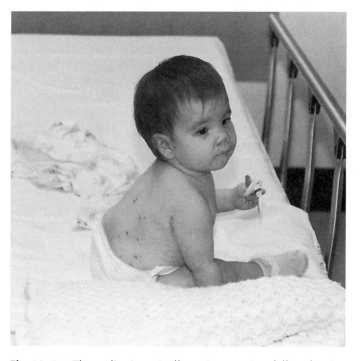

Fig. 10–1   The pediatric varicella patient requires full evaluation for secondary complications.

using acetone (nail polish remover), an ED visit may be
avoided, but this type of situation should be dealt with in compliance with department policies and procedures.

TRIAGE HISTORY

According to the guidelines for analyzing a symptom, the patient with a chief complaint involving the integument is interviewed. The time and manner of onset are particularly important
when forming a conclusion about infection or systemic implications relevant to the patient's presentation. Closed-ended
questions regarding precipitating factors should include questions about the patient's use of hygiene products, exposure to
chemicals or other potential allergens, exposure to other individuals at home or work who have infectious diseases, and the
use of new clothing or other items contacting the patient's integument. The patient should be asked whether others in close
association with them have also complained of similar symptoms or sought medical attention and been diagnosed as having
a dermatology or integument problem in the recent past. Qual-
itative factors relevant to integument symptoms can typically
be obtained by asking patients to explain exactly how they feel.
Radiation and location of integument problems are keys to diagnosis by the physician and should be recorded in triage. The
severity of integument symptoms can be determined by asking
patients just how bad they feel but may also be judged by the
level of interference the patient's symptoms are causing in
regard to sleep, work, and participation in recreation activities.
It is important with pediatric patients to question the historian
about interference of the patient's symptoms with her/his play
and mood. Time factors that should be investigated include the
duration since onset of the symptom, as well as whether the
symptoms are worse at night, during the day, or at noticeable
times or intervals. If the patient has an injury that has caused
him/her to seek ED care, the patient should be asked about first
aid and use of any treatments since the time of the injury.

Determination of the patient's risk for infectious disease
should be carefully considered during the triage assessment. All
patients who are potentially infectious should be isolated from
other patients and families in the waiting area and placed in a

waiting cubicle or ED room with negative airflow or an area considered appropriate for isolation. All health care providers should be notified about the patient's potential contagiousness so that personnel who may be at high risk for infection because of immunosuppression or pregnancy can use protective equipment while caring for the patient.

The triage nurse should ask about the immune status of the patient, and all patients who are immunocompromised should

---

BOX 10–1	**Key Questions To Ask Patients With Problems in the Integument**

- When did you notice the problem?
- How did it start? Suddenly? Gradually? Be specific.
- Do you have any ideas about what may have brought the problem on?
- If the patient has a rash, ask about the patient's medications, use of hygiene products, exposure to allergens, self-administration of narcotics or street drugs, and infection and the health of others with whom the patient is in close association.
- If the patient has received a laceration or has an ecchymosis or injury-associated lesions, ask about the type of injury (penetrating or blunt) and the specific mechanism and conditions of the injury.
- Can you describe how your problem makes you feel? Be as exact as possible.
- Can you point out the exact area of the problem and describe where else you are experiencing the problem?
- Does the problem interfere with your life in any way (sleeping, working, in recreational activities, and so forth)?
- What are the time elements involved in the problem? Do you experience the problem constantly? Does it come and go? Do you notice any associations that you feel are important between your problem and time factors?
- What have you done to make the problem better? If the patient has an injury, ask about the use of first aid and have the patient describe exactly what was done regarding bandaging, ice, and so forth. If the patient has a rash, ask about the use of prescription and nonprescription creams, lotions, and home remedies.
- Have you traveled in the last 12 months? If so, where?

---

be considered for reverse isolation. The triage nurse should also consider the triage designation carefully in patients who are immunocompromised, since problems that are serious in those not compromised may be life threatening in the immunocompromised patient. For example, pediatric patients who are immunosuppressed as a result of cancer or acquired immunodeficiency syndrome (AIDS) are reported to have a higher mortality rate from measles than normal patients, and the illness in some AIDS patients was present without a rash (Kaplan et al., 1992).

All patients with signs and symptoms of infectious illness (particularly, high fever, severe headache, rash, or malaise) should be queried about whether they have traveled in the last 12 months. If so, the triage nurse should find out where the patient has traveled. Problems that are not endemic in the United States are common in other parts of the world where vector-borne diseases such as dengue fever and malaria are carried by mosquitoes. Travelers may become infected during travel without being aware of their illness in its early stages; there were 102 known cases of dengue fever in the United States in 1990 alone (Lange et al., 1992).

All patients with skin breaks resultant from trauma should be asked about the status of their vaccination against tetanus. Any patients who have not had a tetanus vaccination for 10 years or more and are at risk for contracting tetanus after a traumatic break in integrity of the skin should receive a tetanus booster—a need highlighted by the triage nurse.

Key questions to ask patients entering triage with a chief complaint of integument problems are listed in Box 10–1.

PHYSICAL ASSESSMENT

Good lighting in the triage area is particularly helpful for accurately evaluating the patient's skin. The integument is inspected for pigmentation, lesion appearance and distribution, and findings associated with inflammation or infection (Box 10–2). Inspection and palpation are often performed together, and other senses, such as the sense of smell, are used by the triage nurse in determining the possibility of infection or inflammation of the patient's tissue.

When cardinal signs of infection are present in soft tissue,

BOX 10–2	**Signs of Inflammation or Infection**

- Erythema
- Edema
- Tenderness
- Warmth or excessive coolness
- Loss of function
- Foul odor
- Purulent discharge

consideration that an underlying deep systemic infectious process is responsible for the patient's signs and symptoms should be given when determining the patient's triage level. Painful, swollen joints of the hand may be the result of an inflammatory condition, but when the patient reports or has signs of trauma, such as a puncture wound from teeth after the patient has hit someone with a closed fist, the triage nurse should consider the possibility of joint or tissue infection and the patient should be classified as urgent, since initiation of parenteral antibiotic therapy should be considered as soon as possible (Lindsey, 1992). Underlying medical conditions such as diabetes also enter into the decision process when a patient with signs of inflammation or infection is assigned a triage level. Diabetics with foot infections require prompt evaluation and should have a high priority for entry into the ED.

Pigmentation is examined for baseline color, even distribution, and deviations. In dark-skinned patients unevenly distributed areas of lighter pigmentation may be indicative of edema, which can be verified by asking the patient whether the area feels swollen. The nurse may confirm suspected areas of edema by palpation. The examiner should record the presence of erythema, cyanosis, and jaundice. When a lesion, lesions, or a rash is discovered, the triage professional should describe the finding concisely, using the characteristics for describing a lesion (Box 10–3).

A ruler must be used to measure lesions accurately (never compare them with items such as coins or fruit), and gloves

BOX 10–3 **Characteristics for Describing a Lesion**

- Primary or secondary (if reference is available or nurse has a strong knowledge base in dermatology; if specific name of the lesion is given [e.g., macule, papule, crust, or scar], it is irrelevant to state that the lesion is primary or secondary)
- Flat or elevated
- Anatomic location and distribution
- Color
- Size or size range in the case of multiple lesions
- Associated symptoms (pruritus, burning, and the like)
- Precipitants

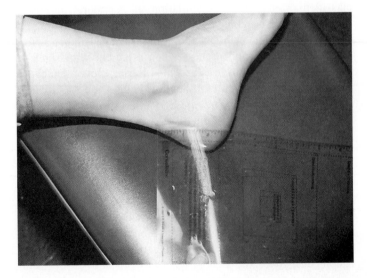

Fig. 10–2 Measurement of skin lesions such as scars should be taken with a clear ruler.

| BOX 10–4 | **Characteristics of Exudate That Should be Recorded** |

- Color
- Odor
- Amount
- Consistency

should be available to the triage nurse for protection from lesions that may be infectious (Fig. 10–2). Masks should also be available to the nurse, since some skin problems are associated with contagious bacterial infections that may be respiratory droplet–borne. If discharge or exudate from a wound, rash, or lesion is present, the nurse should describe it (Box 10–4).

If there is a copious amount of discharge, the triage nurse should apply a nonstick temporary dressing until the patient is examined in the ED.

Most anaphylactic reactions occur within an hour of exposure, although some happen up to 2 days later (Carroll, 1994). Possible manifestations of anaphylaxis include urticaria, angioedema (circumoral and at an extremity, e.g., hands), laryngeal edema, bronchospasm, cardiovascular changes such as tachycardia, gastrointestinal upset, and psychologic distress (fear, panic, or feeling of impending doom). Do not mistake anaphylaxis for a vasovagal reaction. "A patient who is experiencing a vasovagal reaction will be pale, diaphoretic, and either bradycardic or in a normal sinus rhythm; a patient who is having an anaphylactic reaction will be flushed, with warm, dry, pruritic skin and rapid pulse" (Carroll, 1994). The patient who is not hypotensive should be allowed to stay in an upright position for comfort in breathing. Assess for bronchospasm and laryngeal edema by auscultating for wheezes, stridor, changes in voice, and diminished aeration. If the patient clearly has an acute allergic response to an allergen, the need for oxygenation should also be assessed and the patient whose breathing is compromised or who is at high risk for anaphylaxis should be triaged immediately for care to an area where emergency drugs and airway equipment are nearby (Carroll, 1994).

Anaphylaxis kills about 2000 people in the United States each year and affects many more. Penicillin is one of the most common reasons patients have anaphylaxis: of 10,000 administrations, one in four results in fatalities from anaphylaxis. Generally the faster the reaction to the antigen, especially when reaction occurs within 30 minutes, the more serious the signs and symptoms (Yuninger, 1992). Immediate determination of recent medication ingestion by patients with signs and symptoms of anaphylaxis is helpful. As many as 40% of patients may have a recurrence of anaphylaxis within 24 hours of the initial anaphylactic episode (Kaiser et al., 1991). Patients who report having received treatment for anaphylaxis within 24 hours who are having a recurrence of symptoms should be triaged immediately for care, and a record of the prior episode of anaphylaxis should be recorded on the triage record.

Palpation of the Integument

Palpation of the skin is performed to evaluate temperature, moisture, texture, edema, and turgor. The examiner uses the dorsum of the hand to palpate for temperature of the patient's skin, since this part of the hand is more sensitive to temperature variations. Consideration for the temperature of the environment and the patient's psychologic state should be given when evaluating the patient's skin temperature. The examiner palpates distally to proximally using bony anatomic landmarks and surfaces to describe findings accurately. When the patient's skin is assessed for moisture, the normal finding the examiner expects is that the skin is dry but not excessively dry. The palmar surfaces of the examiner's hands are used when palpating the patient's skin for moisture. Diaphoresis or exudate discovered during palpation should be recorded. The normal texture of the skin is smooth, although roughness is often felt over high-trauma surfaces such as the elbows, heels, or knees. Assessment for edema should be performed over any area where inflammation or infection is suspected, as well as over bony prominences of an extremity or portion of an extremity that may look swollen to the examiner.

Skin turgor is most often integrated into the physical assessment of the patient in triage when dehydration or fluid excess is suspected. Pinching a portion of the patient's skin and holding it upward, the examiner allows the skin to fall to its normal anatomic location. If the skin is delayed in returning (anything less than immediate return is considered delayed), "tenting" or "delayed turgor" is noted and the finding recorded on the patient's chart. The best place to evaluate turgor

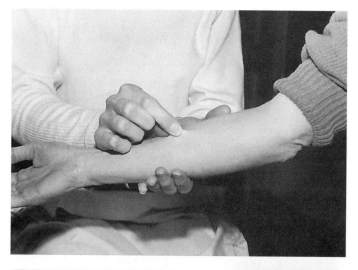

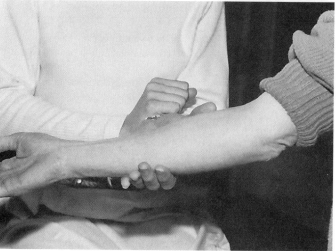

Fig. 10–3 Skin turgor should be evaluated in the adult patient.

in the adult patient is on the forearm, sternum, or forehead, since skin over the patient's dorsal hand, for example, may be highly elastic because of aging. The best place to evaluate the infant's skin turgor is over the abdomen. If the examiner is unable to assess the patient's turgor because of excessively taut skin, this

---

BOX 10–5	**Triage Physical Assessment of the Integument**

- Inspect pigmentation for baseline color and even distribution.
- Inspect for color changes such as pallor, cyanosis, jaundice.
- Inspect and describe lesions and rashes according to characteristics for describing a lesion.
- Inspect for signs of inflammation or infection.
- Palpate for moisture, temperature, edema, texture, and turgor.
- Assess oxygenation need in the case of anaphylaxis or severe allergic response.

BOX 10–6	**Indications for Emergent Triage to ED Care for Integument Problems**

- Vascular lesions (e.g., petechiae or multiple ecchymoses) associated with systemic infections, coagulation disorders, or trauma
- Lacerations associated with nerve damage or interruption of arterial blood flow
- Amputation
- Bites with extensive tissue damage or venom
- Cellulitis over a high-risk area (e.g., face or periorbital area)
- Lesions in association with acute allergic reaction symptoms (e.g., hives, dyspnea, or pulse oximetry <90%)
- Burns associated with acute, severe pain or tissue damage or both
- Burns over high-risk areas (sensory organ or genitalia)
- Congregate symptoms raising suspicion for toxic shock syndrome or group A beta-hemolytic streptococcus
- Anaphylaxis

finding should be recorded as "unable to assess for turgor" and close examination for edema should be performed (Fig. 10–3).

Physical assessment techniques to be used in evaluating the patient's integument are summarized in Box 10–5.

Reasons for an emergent triage designation for ED care of integument problems are listed in Box 10–6.

RASHES

Rashes should be evaluated, however briefly, immediately on the patient's arrival at triage, to determine whether the patient is having an acute allergic response, a systemic allergic reaction, or an infection that may be contagious to others. Pediatric rashes may be caused by a variety of sources, including bacteria, parasites, allergens, and viruses (Campbell, 1993). Although most rashes are minor, some cue conditions requiring emergency treatment. Whether the patient is having an acute allergic response can be determined by asking the patient when the rash appeared, what the patient thinks may have precipitated the rash, and whether the patient has any history of allergic reactions. Of course, some patients have an allergic response to unknown allergens and do not have a history of allergic reactions, but the interviewer's index of suspicion is greater for those patients with a suspected history coupled with a rash that appears to be indicative of an allergic reaction.

Two common "rashes" may be seen in the presence of an acute systemic allergic response to allergens. Wheals (also known as hives or urticaria) may appear, which are linear or circular, pink around the borders, and lighter in the edematous center. Patients often complain of burning or itching when they have hives. All patients with wheals should be asked whether they are able to breathe comfortably; even in the absence of dyspnea the nurse should auscultate the patient's lung fields for airflow and adventitious breath sounds such as wheezing. The second type of rash commonly seen in association with a systemic allergic response is a generalized erythematous rash widely distributed over the body. Again, the patient's airway and breathing must be assessed for compromise and the patient triaged for immediate care if airway, breathing, or circulatory integrity is compromised. Patients with a known history of allergic reactions who carry an EpiPen should be asked whether the kit was used on exposure to the allergen (usually bee sting). Stings from bees, yellow jackets, hornets, wasps, and the like result in 40 deaths per year. Any patient who reports that he/she is allergic to bees and has been stung should be triaged as emergent (Atkinson and Kaliner, 1992). If the patient has a reaction to bee sting or has had a bee sting or another insect sting, the examiner should determine whether the stinger is still in the patient. If ED policy so indicates, the stinger should be removed, following the outlined policy for this practice. Ice should also be applied to the area to minimize the localized inflammatory response.

Description and Classification of Lesions and Rashes

Rashes not suspected to be allergic in origin should be evaluated and described according to the characteristics for describing a lesion. Primary lesions are classified according to size and surface characteristics. Specific descriptors may be used if the examiner is familiar with the terminology and comfortable applying the terms (Box 10–7).

Additional descriptors for describing a lesion may include texture of the lesion, pattern of arrangement, and surface characteristics. These descriptions may be added in the treatment area if necessary.

Secondary lesions are described according to their type, size, and other defining characteristics used for describing a lesion. Secondary lesions are lesions that were initiated with a primary change (e.g., crust or scar). It is important to record secondary lesions when they have relevance to the patient's chief complaint or may have significance to the patient's baseline assessment.

It is not practical to expect that every scar a patient has must be examined, but when the chief complaint is related to skin integrity or a scar is discovered during the assessment in an area where the patient is complaining of discomfort, it is helpful to record the presence of the scar because of the potential for underlying problems. Each scar the nurse identifies may further be described by color, which is useful in determining the age of the scar. In most cases, a scar is closest to baseline pigmentation as it ages. A scar may also be described by size measured in centimeters or millimeters, sur-

---

BOX 10–7	**Primary Lesions**

MACULE

Flat, color-change lesion <1 cm (e.g., freckle)

PATCH

Flat lesion >1 cm (e.g., birthmark)

PAPULE

Elevated, solid lesion <1 cm (e.g., small bug bite)

NODULE

Elevated, solid lesion 1 cm to 2 cm (e.g., ganglion)

TUMOR

Elevated, solid lesion >2 cm (e.g., tumor of any type)

VESICLE

Elevated, fluid-filled lesion <1 cm (e.g., blister)

BULLA

Elevated, fluid-filled lesion >1 cm (e.g., pemphigus)

PUSTULE

Elevated, pus-filled lesion (e.g., acne)

WHEAL

Elevated lesion with erythematous or pink borders, light center (e.g., hives)

---

face characteristics (flat, hypertrophied, atrophied, or keloid), and shape.

Secondary lesions that are sometimes observed and must be described include those that occur as a result of skin breakdown, for example, fissure, erosion, or ulcer. When skin breakdown is observed, the degree of the breakdown and type of surface changes should be recorded and a more extensive classification of the problem and description performed during ED care. Common secondary lesions are listed in Box 10–8.

BOX 10-8 | **Secondary Lesions**

PLAQUE
Coalesced wheals

CRUST
Crusted lesion that was primary originally

SCAR
May be hypertrophied, atrophied, or keloid; describe surface
 characteristics: size, location, color, and shape

FISSURE
Linear crack in epidermis; small, deep, red, or hyperpigmented
 (e.g., cracks at the angles of the mouth)

EROSION
Depressed, moist surface change affecting the epidermis (e.g.,
 following break of vesicle as in chicken pox)

ULCER
Hollowing of epidermis and dermis, red or red-blue (e.g., decubiti)

If a medical diagnosis has already been made of the patient's integument problem, the triage nurse should record the
patient's statement of his/her diagnosis and chief complaint in
quotation marks. For example, if a patient has an erythematous,
maculopapular, linear rash over both forearms in a 7-cm area
and had a diagnosis of scabies 24 hours before arrival at the
ED, the chart reads, "CC: uncontrolled itching" with a secondary note, "I was diagnosed with scabies yesterday at City
Clinic." Of course, all other sections of the triage record, for
example, medications, are completed as usual.

VASCULAR LESIONS

Vascular lesions may be indicative of trauma or systemic problems such as clotting disorders, leukemia, or infectious processes such as bacterial meningitis. Observation of vascular

lesions should include assessment of color, individual size or range, anatomic location, and distribution. Anatomic figures are useful in charting the location and distribution of all lesions, including vascular lesions. Assessment of vascular lesions may be useful in considering reliability of the informant when comparing the age and presentation of injury- or trauma-precipitated vascular lesions with the given history. Location and distribution of lesions may be helpful in determining the index of suspicion for child abuse or domestic violence. If the triage nurse finds a pattern of injuries associated with violence, such as finger imprints or cigarette burns, the patient should be triaged as emergent for care and the safety of the patient and family should be secured. The estimated number of child abuse cases ranges from 50,000 to 70,000 per year (Sheehy, 1990). Estimations of the number of battered women in the United States approach 6 million. These women often seek care for their injuries in EDs, although they are often unlikely to report the actual mechanism and circumstance of their injury (Henderson, 1992). The triage nurse must be informed about the patterns of injuries often associated with abuse so that she/he can be intuitive and inclusive in the triage history and physical. Indications that a patient may be a victim of violence are given in Box 10–9.

Ecchymoses are the most common vascular lesions, and they most often occur in association with traumatic injury. The triage nurse should record the color, size, and location of ecchymoses. The color of the ecchymoses should be recorded, to indicate the age of the injury. Ecchymoses yellow as the time from the tissue insult increases. When ''pattern'' ecchymoses are present (e.g., in the shape of fingers or a hand), this should be indicated. Ecchymoses of varying ages and in locations not typically associated with accidental trauma, such as over the back, chest, and abdomen, are a particularly critical presentation, since this pattern is commonly seen in victims of abuse such as child abuse victims or battered women or men. Appropriate agencies should be notified when abuse of any type is suspected. Ecchymoses not associated with known trauma may indicate an underlying hematologic problem. In patients whose chief complaint relates to unexplained or excessive ecchymoses, orthostatic vital signs should be assessed and tolerance to orthostatic changes should also be recorded.

BOX 10-9	**Indications That a Patient May Be a Victim of Violence**

- Delay in seeking care
- Changing history regarding the mechanism and situation of injury or evasiveness or refusal to provide information
- Listless or fearful affect
- Refusal of possible perpetrator to leave patient alone with triage nurse or other health care provider while the patient is interviewed or examined
- Possible perpetrator directing anger toward patient or showing little concern for the patient's well-being or injuries
- Unusual injuries such as cigarette burns, human bites, perineal injuries
- Height and weight grossly disproportionate
- Injuries over areas not in concert with reported history of event (e.g., ecchymoses over the back)
- Fingerprint ecchymoses
- Frequent, multiple injuries or use of the emergency department for nonspecific problems

---

Purpura is a rare vascular lesion that is purple to purple-red and is localized or generalized throughout the body. Sometimes seen in association with untoward drug reactions, purpuric lesions may herald a critical side effect of medication. Because they are uncommon and are possibly associated with life-threatening drug reactions or acute leukemia or thrombocytopenia, all patients with this type of lesion should be triaged as emergent (Rosen, 1992). In children purpuric lesions have been seen in association with meningococcemia (Holland et al., 1993), although petechiae are more common in this infection.

Petechiae are red, pinpoint hemorrhages that occur in association with tissue trauma or may be signs of bacterial meningitis (Fig. 10-4). Again, because of the critical associations with life-threatening illnesses, all patients with petechiae, whether localized or generalized, should be triaged as needing immediate care. If the patient is febrile and has signs of meningitis, personnel should be alert to the benefits of having individuals exposed to the patient's respiratory droplets wear

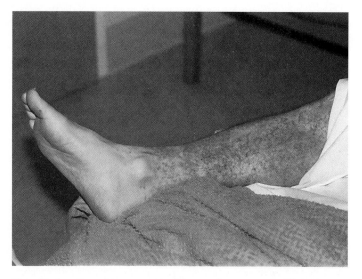

Fig. 10–4   Petechiae seen in triage of an acutely ill leukemic patient.

masks to keep from contracting the bacterial infection causing the meningitis. Bacterial meningitis can be lethal within hours, and patients with this problem benefit from early detection and emergent triage for aggressive, immediate care.

Vascular lesions that may be evident in examining the patient's integument but are not of critical importance include spider angiomas, venous stars, telangiectasias, and capillary hemangiomas. Patients with complaints related to these lesions may be triaged as nonurgent in most cases. However, as with capillary hemangiomas in some children, there is interruption of airway patency caused by internal lesions. Significant vascular lesions that may be seen in triage are described in Box 10–10.

SPECIFIC SKIN DISORDERS
Cellulitis

Cellulitis is a common skin problem resulting in inflammatory color changes. It is often a result of tissue infection. Precipi-

BOX 10–10	**Vascular Lesions of Particular Significance in Triage**

ECCHYMOSES

Discoloration; various shades of red; yellow as time since onset increases; variable size; precipitated by destruction of the vascular wall, trauma, inflammatory processes

HEMATOMA

Red-purple or skin-toned initially in some patients; elevated; varying in size; resulting from collection of extravasated blood contained in the tissues of the skin, which is precipitated by trauma or incomplete hemostasis after an invasive procedure or surgery

PURPURA

Red-purple discoloration that does not blanch, >0.5 cm, precipitated by intravascular defects or infection

PETECHIAE

Red-purple discoloration that does not blanch, <0.5 cm, precipitated by intravascular defects, infection

---

tating factors may be clearly stated, for example, bug bite or use of dirty needles for intravenous drug use, or they may be unknown. Cellulitis is most often caused by streptococcal or staphylococcal organisms. This form of tissue infection may be life threatening or may cause extensive, permanent tissue damage if unrecognized and untreated. The skin is erythematous or hyperpigmented in the dark-skinned patient and hot to touch, and may be abnormal over a wide area or in streaks. Enlarged lymph nodes near the infected area may be palpable. Patients with cellulitis should have a minimum triage designation of "urgent."

Indications that the patient must be triaged as emergent include cases of group A beta-hemolytic streptococcus (GABHS) sepsis with a rapid, fulminant course that mimics the presentation of staphylococcal toxic shock. Frequently the sepsis begins with an infection in the skin or soft tissue that is associated with fever, rash, desquamation, hypotension, and multiple–organ system dysfunction (Wood et al., 1993). Any patient with elements of this life-threatening problem should be triaged as emergent for immediate care.

Lesions Common to Drug-Addicted Patients

Skin lesions in patients who intravenously self-administer street drugs or narcotics are easily identified by most ED personnel and often are voluntarily identified by the patient. In intravenous drug users "track marks" are commonly seen in the antecubital fossa and dorsa of the hands but may also be seen in remote areas such as the feet and, occasionally, the breasts of pregnant women because of the dilated condition of the vessels and easy access for drug administration. Thus it is important for all patients with sepsis or chief complaints involving the integument to be entirely disrobed once they are in the ED for care. Abscesses and scars caused by old abscesses and tracks are commonly visible in intravenous drug users and are accentuated by hyperpigmentation in sun-exposed areas. Ulcerations are not unusual in patients who abuse pentazocine (Talwin) and methamphetamine ("crystal"). Other symptoms such as urticaria, pruritus, and excoriations are commonly associated with drugs that release histamine (Rosen, 1992). Areas where the skin has been picked or scratched may be seen in the children of drug and alcohol abusers.

Erythema Multiforme

It is not uncommon for ED personnel to see erythema multiforme, which appears as a "rash" with plaques on the trunk and extremities that have a characteristic target appearance with mucosal involvement in one third of patients. Typically thought of as an adolescent problem, erythema multiforme may also occur in young children and adults of any age. Erythema multiforme may be precipitated by drugs such as sulfonamides, penicillins, phenylbutazone and phenytoin, and methotrexate. Drug-induced erythema multiforme causes the majority of life-threatening forms of this integument disorder. Other causes of eruptions include herpes simplex and mycoplasmic infection. The triage nurse should be familiar with the risk factors for and appearance of this rash because, although it is a minor problem in many patients, it may be a severe, life-threatening problem when respiratory structures and the esophagus are involved (Stampien and Schwartz, 1992).

Pruritus

Itching may be associated with common skin problems such as eczema, dermatitis, or scabies, but it may occur in association with or as a prodrome to serious health problems such as Hodgkin's disease and many other cancers and medical problems (Rosen, 1992). Knowing this, triage nurses should seriously concern themselves with taking a few moments to ask patients about their general health. Helpful information that may also be gleaned during the triage interview of the patient with pruritus includes bathing practices and the presence of medical conditions commonly associated with pruritus such as diabetes mellitus, renal failure, polycythemia vera, and AIDS (Klecz and Schwartz, 1992). The triage nurse should encourage patients to follow up with their regular health care provider once their emergency evaluation and care have been completed. Followup care is taught in detail by the ED care providers, but it is not too early to introduce the importance of follow-up in the triage area, since this is the patient's first introduction to ED care and concern by the triage nurse about the patient's long-term wellbeing encourages compliance.

Integumentary Manifestations of AIDS

Nearly every patient with human immunodeficiency virus (HIV) at some time has a skin disorder. This may be the first indication of HIV infection. The five major categories of disorders are bacterial, fungal, protozoal, viral, and neoplastic (Anastasi and Rivera, 1992). With the high incidence of AIDS in the United States the triage nurse is well advised to be familiar with the characteristic appearance of these infections for early identification of the patient who may have an AIDS-related complication of the integument.

COMMONLY TREATED RASHES

Rash illnesses are difficult to diagnose in many cases. It is not the role of the triage professional to diagnose, but it is helpful for infection-related problems to be identified early to prevent spread of infection to other individuals in the waiting area. Infection-related or contagious rash problems and illnesses that may become evident in the emergency setting include (but are not limited to) measles, chicken pox, impetigo, scabies, and bacterial meningitis (see Vascular Lesions). When any contagious illness is suspected, the patient should be asked about known exposure to others (family, friends, children in day care, and so forth) with known infectious disease. Common skin rashes with potential for contagion are presented in Table 10–1.

All patients with suspected contagious illnesses should be isolated from others until contagiousness is disproved. Some patients request medical care for "an infection," which they indicate by showing a rash to the triage nurse. The triage nurse should enter the chief complaint as "rash," then quote the patient's concern.

Table 10–1 Common Skin Rashes With Contagion Potential

Problem	Rash characteristics	Associated signs and symptoms
Measles	Generalized, papular, red	Koplik's spots in mouth; runny nose, light sensitivity, fever, pruritus
Chicken pox (varicella)	Vesicular with crusting lesions in various stages; generalized	Runny nose, fever, cough, pruritus
Impetigo	Vesicular with crusting over erythematous base; localized initially, then spreading	
Scabies	Maculopapular, linear rash often between the fingers, at the neck, and on forearms but may be atypical	Severe, persistent pruritus

All patients with rash, particularly in the summer, should be asked about the possibility of tick bite. Rocky Mountain spotted fever, although rare in some parts of the country, may be life threatening. It is precipitated by tick bite and followed by a rash; 10% of rashes begin on the trunk in children (Simon, 1992). Lyme disease is another potentially devastating complication of a tick bite that may occur anywhere from 3 to 30 days after a tick bite from an infected tick. Characteristics of Lyme disease are a bull's eye–appearing rash, with occasional accompaniment of other symptoms such as fever, headache, neck pain, myalgia, and nausea (Masters, 1993).

Pediatric patients with diaper rash may have dermatitis, yeast infection, or other infectious rashes (Farrington, 1992). The triage nurse should be familiar with the common causes of diaper rashes so that he/she might begin education, as time permits, of the patient regarding care of the infant.

Herpes Zoster

Herpes zoster, or "shingles," commonly occurs as a localized vesicular rash that follows a dermatome. This can be a serious problem and may cause blindness when the facial nerve is involved. Triage nurses should be alert to the fact that not all patients have the characteristic dermatomal rash and pain. Some have radicular pain without an eruption (Gilden et al., 1992). These patients should be classified as urgent and not triaged for clinic or primary provider care unless they can be immediately seen for evaluation and comfort measures. Patients who are immunosuppressed are at a higher risk for herpes zoster.

Some patients do have skin problems indicative of infection, such as candidiasis of the mouth ("thrush") or buttocks, which is common in patients with cancer or AIDS and in children receiving antibiotics, but the infection is not contagious so the patient does not need to be isolated. If the triage professional does not have a strong background in dermatology or in the recognition of contagious diseases or the ability to easily discern patients who require isolation, it is better to confer with the charge nurse or, if necessary, err on the side of caution.

Rashes common in the general population requesting medical or nursing attention include contact dermatitis and eczema. These patients usually have a history of prior outbreaks and report precipitants that have exacerbated the skin problem. The condition is not urgent in most cases, so nonurgent designation and potential triage to care in a clinic or from a private physician are often appropriate. Even when a patient has not had prior episodes of dermatitis or eczema, if there is a low index of suspicion for infectious processes, the patient may be triaged away from emergency services for care. Primary care for chronic, nonurgent skin conditions is most helpful for patients, since identification of possible allergens and continuity of follow-up care are available.

LACERATIONS AND TRAUMATIC LESIONS SUCH AS SNAKE BITE AND AMPUTATION

All patients with traumatic tissue breaks who enter triage require nursing intervention that is concurrent with an assessment of the tissue trauma. Furthermore, for every patient with a chief complaint of traumatic tissue breaks, tetanus immunization status should be determined and infection potential minimized.

Lacerations should be evaluated in triage for size, avulsion, and extent of tissue damage (e.g., superficial), and location. The object or event precipitating the break in tissue integrity should be determined during the interview, as well as initial first aid applied by the patient. The patient's sensation around the laceration should be assessed to evaluate for nerve damage, which would cause the triage designation to be upgraded from urgent to emergent. All patients should have neurovascular checks distal and proximal to a wound to determine the presence of circulatory compromise (Fig. 10–5). Lacerations should be fully exposed to the triage nurse for assessment unless bleeding is controlled by the dressing. If tissues or paper products have been used to dress the wound, these should be removed and the area lightly rinsed with normal saline solution. Temporary dressings should be of nonstick material and applied to control bleeding. Care should be taken to prevent impairment of circulation. Patients with lacerations or crush injuries that have resulted in amputation of a digit or body part should be triaged as emergent. If the patient has entered the emergency system without the severed part, significant others or family accompanying the patient should be sent to retrieve the part if possible. When crush injuries occur, it is unlikely that reattachment will

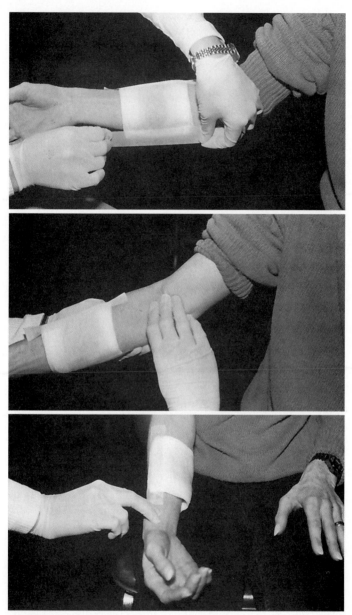

Fig. 10–5 A temporary dressing is applied before assessment of brachial and radial pulses, proximal and distal to the injury site.

be attempted, but the possibility may exist and it is better to have the part. A sterile cup containing a small amount of crushed ice should be provided; the severed part will be placed on the ice in the sterile cup. Direct contact between a severed part and ice should be avoided to prevent frostbite of the severed tissue. The triage professional should not have a patient with a laceration soak the injured area in normal saline or any other solution in an attempt to prevent tissue maceration and swelling because the soaking renders the tissue boggy and difficult to work with during reattachment.

Patients who enter the triage area with a chief complaint of having been bitten should be interviewed immediately. The human bite that causes a break in tissue integrity may lead to serious tissue infections. Even when the patient is not in acute distress, this patient should be triaged as "urgent." Bites from dogs, cats, or other pets should be cleaned thoroughly as soon after the bite as possible, and the patient should be triaged as "urgent" unless tissue damage is severe and extensive (Fig. 10–6). The patient's tetanus immunization status should be de-

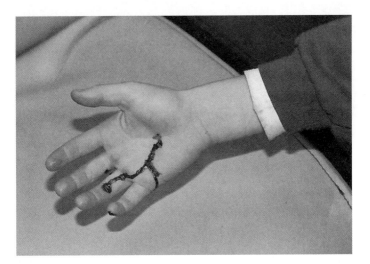

Fig. 10–6 A dog bite laceration should be assessed and then cleansed with normal saline in triage. Tetanus status must always be determined.

termined, and information regarding whether the bite was un-provoked should also be recorded in the patient history. If the status of vaccinations in the dog or cat is known, it is also helpful to record this information. In general, animal bites must be reported to animal control.

Bites caused by snakes or reptiles should be evaluated im-mediately, and a determination made, if possible, concerning what specific reptile caused the bite and whether it had ven-omous potential. Occasionally patients enter triage with the of-fending reptile bagged for inspection. Examination of potentially poisonous reptiles is not the role of the triage nurse and should be deferred. Twenty-five percent of snake bites cause envenomation. If the potential of a poisonous snake bite is present, the patient's extremity or part that was bitten should be immobilized and the patient should be kept quiet and triaged emergently for care.

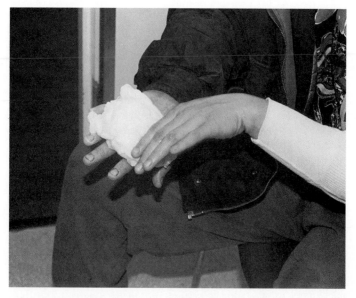

Fig. 10–7   Chemical burns to the hands are treated in triage with cool saline dressings for comfort.

BURNS

In the triage area patients who enter with a chief complaint of a burn usually receive their triage interview and assessment immediately on arriving for care. If policy dictates, the triage nurse determines the exact extent of the burns using as a guide the rule of nines or the degree of the burns. Any patient with severe pain whose burns are more than superficial and small, especially those with burns over high-risk areas such as the face or genitalia or involving respiratory structures, should be triaged as emergent and instructed to take nothing by mouth until otherwise instructed. It is helpful for the triage professional to identify the cause of the burn (heat, electricity, chemicals, radiation, or gases), what initial treatment may have been instituted (cool water, grease, or the like), and the time of the injury. If ED care is delayed, treatment in triage should include immobilization of

---

| BOX 10–11 | **Triage Nursing Interventions for Problems in the Integument** |

LACERATION

Superficial cleansing with normal saline solution and light, bulky dressing unless bleeding is not controlled, in which case pressure dressing may be necessary

INJURY-ASSOCIATED EDEMA, PAIN

Application of ice, elevation, compression, and immobilization as indicated by triage nurse's judgment and with consideration for the possibility of compartment syndrome or neurovascular complications associated with injury

RASH ILLNESS

Isolation of patients with potential for infection, application of light dressing if copious exudate exists

PARTIAL-THICKNESS BURN

Cool saline basin

SNAKE BITE

Rest and elevation of affected extremity

---

the affected area; a light, sterile, dry dressing; and supportive communication (Fig. 10–7). Patients whose burns have caused blistering should be told not to rupture the blisters, since rupture may lead to infection. Patients who do not complain of pain but whose burns are more extensive than simple erythema may have whole skin loss to deep tissue loss and require immediate treatment. When any individual has received a burn as a result of violence, this information should be shared with the appropriate agencies.

NURSING INTERVENTIONS IN TRIAGE

First aid should be administered with the permission of the patient as needed for all rashes, lesions, lacerations, and burns. Comfort measures should be initiated as swiftly as possible, to effectively reduce the patient's long-range need for pain relief measures. Nursing interventions for problems in the integument are given in Box 10–11.

REFERENCES

Anastasi JK, Rivera J: Skin manifestations of H.I.V., *Nursing* 22(11):55, 1992.

Atkinson TP, Kaliner MA: Anaphylaxis, *Med Clin North Am* 76(4):841, 1992.

Campbell LS: Assessing pediatric rashes, *RN* 56(4):59, 1993.

Carroll R: Speed: the essential response to anaphylaxis, *RN* 57(6):26, 1994.

Cowan M et al: Serious group A beta-hemolytic streptococcal infections complicating varicella, *Ann Emerg Med* 23(4):818, 1994.

Farrington E: Diaper dermatitis, *Pediatr Nurs* 18(1):81, 1992.

Gilden D et al: Varicella-zoster virus reactivation without rash, *J Infect Dis* 166(Suppl 1):S30, 1992.

Henderson A: Critical care nurses need to know about abused women, *Crit Care Nurse* 12(2):27, 1992.

Holland J et al: Nursing care of a child with meningococcemia, *J Pediatr Nurs* 8(4):211, 1993.

Kaiser HB, Kaliner MA, Scott JL: Anaphylaxis: when routine turns nightmare, *Patient Care* 25(9):16, 1991.

Kaplan L et al: Severe measles in immunocompromised patients, *JAMA* 267(9):1237, 1992.

Klecz R, Schwartz R: Pruritus, *Am Fam Physician* 45(6):2681, 1992.

Lange R, Beall B, Denny S: Dengue fever: a resurgent risk for the international traveler, *Am Fam Physician* 45(3):1161, 1992.

Lindsey D: Soft tissue infections, *Emerg Med Clin North Am* 10(4):737, 1992.

Masters E: Erythema migrans: rash as key to early diagnosis of Lyme disease, *Postgrad Med* 94(1):133, 137, 1993.

Rosen P et al: *Emergency medicine: concepts and clinical practice,* ed 3, St Louis, 1992, Mosby.

Sheehy S: *Mosby's manual of emergency care,* St Louis, 1990, Mosby.

Simon J: Computerized diagnostic referencing in pediatric emergency medicine, *Pediatr Clin North Am* 39(5):1165, 1992.

Stampien T, Schwartz R: Erythema multiforme, *Am Fam Physician* 46(4):1171, 1992.

Wood T, Potter M, Jonasson O: Streptococcal toxic shock–like syndrome: the importance of surgical intervention, *Ann Surg* 217(2):109, 1993.

Yuninger JW: Anaphylaxis, *Ann Allergy* 69(2):87, 1992.

RECOMMENDED READING

Brady W, DeBehnke D, Crosby D: Dermatological emergencies, *Am J Emerg Med* 12(2):217, 1994.

Fitzpatrick T et al, eds: *Dermatology in general medicine: textbook and atlas,* ed 4, 2 vols, New York, 1993, McGraw-Hill.

11 Problems With Invasive Medical Equipment

Many patients who live in the community have invasive devices previously used only in hospitalized patients. After surgery, patients are discharged from inpatient hospital settings earlier and with a higher level of acuity than in the past. Many patients in the community need equipment that drains body fluids or provides nutrition and fluids that cannot be ingested through a natural route.

Patients who have intravenous lines (IVs) and tubes inserted for medical purposes often have a sophisticated familiarity with their equipment that enables them to successfully troubleshoot many problems. Resource personnel such as enterostomal nurses or IV therapy nurses are often available through home health agencies, public health departments, or hospital outpatient services. These specialists are helpful to patients dealing with problems related to their medical equipment or health. Resource personnel are identified for the community health care patient when the patient is discharged and should be the first persons the patient calls if an equipment malfunction occurs. When resource personnel are unavailable, patients with medical equipment or health crises may seek emergency services for care. At times, patients have normally functioning invasive equipment but require emergency services for other reasons.

It is helpful and important for triage professionals to be familiar with the types of invasive equipment commonly seen in community health care and to understand the acuity of common equipment problems that may arise, to triage and treat "equipped" patients appropriately.

CENTRAL VENOUS LINES

Central IV lines are used in acute-care patients who require careful hemodynamic monitoring, temporary pacemakers, or large-volume fluid replacement (Figs. 11–1 and 11–2). Another

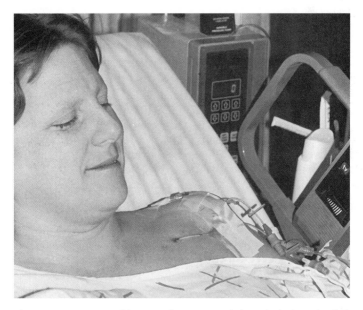

Fig. 11–1 A central line is often inserted directly below the left clavicle.

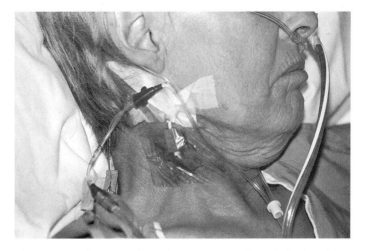

Fig. 11–2 The internal jugular vein is a preferred site for placement of a central line.

BOX 11–1	Common Indications for a Central Venous Line in Outpatients

- Administration of total parenteral nutrition or hypertonic solutions
- Easy access for frequent blood drawing
- Lack of peripheral intravenous (IV) sites when fluids or medications must be administered intravenously
- Access for administration of medications that are most safely given through a central line
- Long-term maintenance therapy

reason for central line placement is the need for central line support in the acute-care patient or the chronically ill or challenged individual. Common indications for central IV lines in community health care patients are listed in Box 11–1.

To understand the potential problems of patients with a central line, it is important for the triage nurse to be familiar with the anatomic placement of central lines, as well as the various types of central lines and how they differ.

Central Venous Line Placement

Placement of central lines is performed using sterile procedure. The jugular vein is usually the first choice for large-volume fluid administration. This site is less likely than other sites to be seen in community-based patients with central lines. Large peripheral veins such as the femoral vein are sometimes selected for central line insertion but are not desirable sites, since the patient may no longer safely bend the extremity where the central line is placed. These veins are used only when other sites are not easily accessible or usable. The right subclavian vein is a straight passage that avoids the thoracic duct. Because this vein has relatively few acute complications associated with insertion, it is often the vessel of choice for acute and long-term needs. Many patients who are known to require a long-term central line have a procedure whereby the subclavian is "tunnel-accessed," which provides occlusion to air and organisms while allowing for central venous access for line placement (Fig. 11–3).

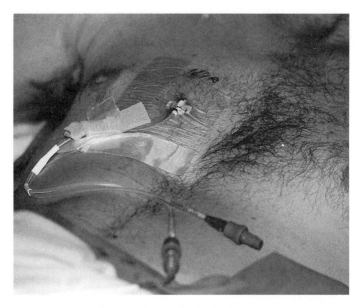

Fig. 11–3 Groshong catheter placed for long-term use in an on-cology patient.

BOX 11–2	**Triage Questions To Ask the Patient With a Central Venous Line**

- What type of central line do you have?
- Why do you have a central line?
- What kinds of fluids and medications are given through your central line?
- Have you had or been treated for any problems with the central line?
- Where is the central line placed?
- How often do you change the dressing over the central line? When was the last time it was changed?
- Do you use antibiotic ointment over the catheter site? Do you flush the catheter with antibiotics?
- Have you noticed any problems with redness, swelling, tenderness, excess drainage, or pus?
- How often do you flush the central line? What do you use to flush it with?

For all patients with central lines fundamental information about their central line must be determined during the triage interview (Box 11–2).

Routine Catheter Care

It is important to ask the patient with a central line about the routine care of the catheter, since, regardless of the number of ports, routine care to prevent complications should be performed. This care should include flushing the catheter to maintain patency, changing the injection cap, cleansing the exit site, and applying a prescribed dressing over the catheter site to prevent infection (Freedman and Bosserman, 1993). The exact specifics of the routine care vary according to the policies and procedures of the supervising physician and the agency responsible for the patient's care, but the fundamental elements should not vary.

Physical Assessment

Physical assessment of the patient with a central line is guided by the history and the general appearance of the patient. Guidelines for physical assessment of a patient with a central line are given in Box 11–3, and the triage nurse will see the rationale for each physical assessment technique used in triage as the complications of central line placement are reviewed.

COMPLICATIONS ASSOCIATED WITH CENTRAL VENOUS LINE PLACEMENT
Short-term Complications

Short-term complications are most often evident in the early phases of the patient's recovery from central line placement and include dysrhythmias resulting from cardiac irritation during the procedure, pneumothorax resulting from pleural nicking, bleeding, hematoma formation, and air embolism. Although these complications are almost always exclusive to the early, postrecovery phase of placement, hematoma formation may be a process that persists slowly during later recovery and causes ensuing complications. Pneumothorax continues to be a risk factor. Surface hematomas are easy to recognize, since a red-purple discoloration of the skin is present and obvious extravasation of blood into the tissues is evident. Unless patients

| BOX 11–3 | **Triage Physical Assessment of Patients With a Central Line** |

Inspect the site for clarity and chart the presence of discharge, edema, erythema, tenderness, or warmth if discovered.

Chart the presence and appearance of sutures.

Inspect the line for kinks in the tubing and integrity of the external tubing.

Palpate for crepitus of the thorax.

Palpate distal peripheral pulses for presence and bilateral equality.

Check hand grips for bilateral and adequate strength.

| BOX 11–4 | **Assessment for Signs of a Pneumothorax** |

ASSESS VITAL SIGNS

Tachypnea, tachycardia

AUSCULTATE FOR BILATERAL BREATH SOUNDS

Diminished or absent breath sounds, asymmetry of breath sounds

PALPATE FOR THORACIC CREPITATION

Subcutaneous crepitation

PALPATE FOR BILATERAL CHEST EXPANSION

Asymmetric expansion of chest

PERFORM PULSE OXIMETRY

Pulse oximetry $<90\%$

complain of persistent pain or infection, they are unlikely to seek emergency care for a surface hematoma. Internal hematomas are not externally evident, however, and the nurse must be astute in recognizing the signs of internal hematomas in patients with vague or unclear complaints related to a central line. As pressure rises from an internal hematoma, vital structures located nearby are affected, and the patient often has numbness and tingling from nerve pressure and, in the "worst case" scenario, diminished or absent pulses distal to the hematoma as arterial occlusion ensues. Therefore, even when hematoma formation is unlikely in the patient with a chronic condition, it is wise to incorporate assessment for peripheral pulses into the triage evaluation of patients with central lines. A neurovascular check should also be performed on the same-side extremity of the central-line catheter.

A pneumothorax that occurs during line placement trauma may not be noticed during the early, postrecovery phase. Patients who are triaged with a chief complaint of chest pain or dyspnea who also have a central line should be assessed for the possibility of a pneumothorax (Box 11–4). Any indication that a pneumothorax exists is cause for immediate concern. Any patient with compromise of respiratory or circulatory functions should be triaged into the emergency department (ED) as emergent.

Long-term Complications

Long-term complications of central lines are legion, although in one study of 1422 patients with permanent venous access devices fewer than 1% of patients had life-threatening complications associated with their equipment (Sariego et al., 1993).

Sepsis. The most common complication associated with long-term central lines is sepsis (Box 11–5).

Some practitioners think that sepsis can be prevented through the use of an antibiotic flush routine using vancomycin (Cowan, 1993), although this procedure is not universal. Antibacterial solutions bonded to the catheter have shown promising results in reducing central venous catheter sepsis in some studies (Orr, 1993). Catheter-related sepsis is common in patients with long-term devices but less common in patients with implanted ports (Groeger et al., 1993). Patients with infection elsewhere are at higher risk for catheter sepsis than are patients who do not have infection. Other risk factors associated with catheter sepsis include inappropriate catheter care, inappropriate duration of catheter use, and hospitalization for more than 14 days (Ena et al., 1992). Catheter sepsis may be caused by a number of other factors, including contamination of intravenous

BOX 11–5	**Signs of Catheter Sepsis or Infection or Both**

- Fever
- Tissue redness
- Swelling
- Warmth
- Tenderness
- Purulent exudate or discharge

---

fluids, contamination during handling of catheter equipment, and migration of bacteria along the subcutaneous insertion path (Orr, 1993). The location of erythema and edema depends on the location and origin of the infection; exit site and tunnel infections cause erythema, tenderness, and induration within 2 cm of catheter exit, and septicemia, septic thrombosis, and port pocket infection cause fever and general signs and symptoms of infection without erythema and edema around the tunnel or exit site (Kitt and Kaiser, 1990). An indication of sepsis in patients receiving parenteral nutrition is hyperglycemia. The patient who has signs and symptoms of hyperglycemia (excessive thirst, urination, and blood sugar level >160 mg/ml) and who is receiving parenteral nutrition via central venous catheter should be evaluated for sepsis (Potter and Perry, 1994). The triage nurse must know that sepsis may be caused by fungi as well as bacteria, although the symptoms will not differ according to the origin of the infection.

The triage nurse, if time permits, should ask patients about their techniques of catheter care and the type, amount, and infusion time of intravenous fluids used. In addition to asking the patient what type of device the patient has, the nurse may ask the patient if she/he knows whether the catheter has been bonded with antibiotics, a technique that has been shown to reduce the incidence of catheter-related sepsis and may be used in patients that are at highest risk for sepsis morbidity and mortality (e.g., patients with acquired immunodeficiency syndrome [AIDS]). Patients with sepsis and tissue swelling may also have dysfunction of the line wherein it becomes occluded. The triage professional must record the history of the patient as well as the physical assessment findings but does not need to verify line dysfunction; that is verified in the ED. If the patient has a fever, the triage nurse should ask about the onset of fever at home, since the probability of bacteremia increases daily in the presence of catheter-related sepsis (Orr, 1993).

Catheter occlusion. Loss of patency of a venous access device or central line may occur as a result of tube kinking, malposition, a fibrin sheath, deposit of lipid (particularly with lipid infusions), tubing malfunction or breakage, or drug precipitates (Orr, 1993). The patient or care provider notices the occlusion when she/he attempts to withdraw blood or infuse fluids. Catheter occlusion may be a result of improper line flushing. Proper line flushing is performed with continuous positive pressure during the last 0.5 ml of flush administration, depending on the type of catheter. With improper flushing, a vacuum forms at the catheter tip, and fibrin formation and occlusion at the internal catheter tip occur.

Patients whose chief complaint is catheter occlusion should have the central line examined for number of available ports (in a multiport system). Catheters may be occluded only during aspiration when the surface of the vein is aspirated into the tip and blood cannot be withdrawn. If blood cannot be aspirated, the nurse should not assume that the catheter is completely malfunctioning, since infusion of fluids may still be possible. A gentle attempt to infuse fluids through a syringe (e.g., 5 ml normal saline solution) allows the nurse to judge whether the occlusion affects withdrawal or withdrawal and infusion.

If all ports are occluded and fluid or medication administration is necessary on an urgent basis, the patient must be triaged as emergent. If the catheter has one or more functioning ports that may be used for fluid or medication administration, the patient may be triaged as nonurgent or urgent, often depending on the patient's condition and reason for visit.

Thrombophlebitis. As in patients with all types of intravenous catheters, thrombophlebitis and thrombotic complications are commonly seen in patients with central lines (Raad et al., 1994). In the absence of fever the catheter site or an area distal to the catheter site may be tender and show other signs of inflammation, such as erythema and edema of the catheter site, surrounding area, or distal locations such as the neck or chest wall. The patient may report poor catheter function. The patient should be triaged as urgent, since the risks of venous thrombosis or thromboembolism are acute in the patient with thrombophlebitis. In one study of cancer patients with implanted venous access devices it was discovered that left-sided ports with catheter tips lying in the upper part of the vena cava were at highest risk for thrombotic complications (Puel et al., 1993), but any patient with signs of thrombosis or thrombophlebitis around a central venous catheter or venous access device should be triaged as emergent for ED care.

Brachial plexus damage. Brachial plexus damage is possible after central line placement. As with a suspected hematoma, it is recommended that, to assess for the possibility of brachial plexus damage, all patients with central lines receive neurovascular checks bilaterally on extremities distal to the central line insertion site. Hand grips should be checked for bilateral and adequate strength.

Extravasation. Extravasation, or leakage of fluids into the tissues, may occur as a result of thrombosis, catheter tip dislocation, catheter damage, or, in implantable ports, dislodgment of the needle and port (Camp-Sorrell, 1992). The level of damage and triage acuity relative to extravasation depends on the type of fluids absorbed into the tissues, particularly if medication is involved. If medication is involved in extravasation, the triage nurse must determine what drug was being infused and when the infusion was initiated. The patient who enters triage with complaints of pain or burning at the pocket of the port or chest or neck pain after the infusion was initiated should have the possibility of extravasation considered (Kitt and Kaiser, 1990). The patient should be triaged for immediate care if antidotes may be effectively administered to counteract tissue damage or if the tissue damage is of a critical degree; emergent triage also ensures initiation of comfort measures such as warm compresses, if indicated, according to the recommendations for the drug involved.

Many complications result in emergent triage to ED care for the patient with a central line. Some of these are listed in Box 11–6.

BOX 11–6	Common Indications for Emergent Triage Designation in Patients With Central Venous Line

COMMON PROBLEMS

Cardiac tamponade, hemothorax, perforation, endocarditis, and air
embolism

SIGNS AND SYMPTOMS

Chest pain, dyspnea, tachycardia, and orthostatic vital signs

INTUITIVE JUDGMENT

Triage nurse or care provider judges that the patient is in crisis

CATHETER TYPES
Short-term Catheters

Percutaneous inserted central catheters (PICCs) and other catheters (Box 11–7) are usually used for patients who require central lines for a relatively short time or for less than 2 weeks.
PICCs are inserted into antecubital veins, can be used long-
term, and may be advisable in patients who cannot tolerate central lines in the neck or chest (Orr, 1993). PICCs are rarely
implicated in catheter-related sepsis; in fact, in one study of
patients with PICC lines, bacteremia did not occur in any patients, and bacterial colonization occurred in only 11 (11%) of
100 patients (Pauley et al., 1993).

Long-term Catheters

Types of central venous lines, including those for long-term use,
are listed in Box 11–7. Implantable ports, for long-term use, are
totally implanted and are often used for patients with breast
cancer, since the devices allow the patient freedom to wear
clothing that may expose the area and also allow the patient to
swim or participate in sports without the concern of external
tubing. Implantable ports must be accessed using a Huber
needle, which is inserted through the skin to enter the port; use
of this device should be indicated on the triage record, since not

---

BOX 11–7	**Types of Central Venous Lines**

SHORT-TERM USE

Percutaneous inserted central catheter
Landmark

LONG-TERM USE

Groshong
Hickman
Broviac
Port-a-Cath
Implantable ports

---

all emergency personnel may be familiar with the device (Potter and Perry, 1994). The latest implantable ports may be found not on the chest but in the antecubital area; these are accessed from the side of the device instead of from the top, also using a Huber needle (Camp-Sorrell, 1992). Complications with long-term catheters are similar to those with any venous access device, such as occlusion and infection. Implanted infusion devices that are not in use must be flushed with heparinized solution every 4 weeks to maintain patency, and patients with an implanted infusion device should be queried about this maintenance requirement, particularly if they complain of occlusion (Potter and Perry, 1994).

NURSING INTERVENTIONS IN TRIAGE

The comfort level a triage nurse has in dealing with central venous lines depends primarily on his/her hands-on experience in working with this type of invasive equipment. All triage nurses might be faced with situations in dealing with central lines that they must act on safely. Questions to ask about central lines are listed in Box 11–8. There are many complications that may arise with central venous catheters, some of which have been discussed in this chapter. Triage nurses who are not quite comfortable in troubleshooting or assessing central venous catheters should request assistance from a colleague who is

BOX 11–8	Triage Questions the Nurse Might Ask About a Central Venous Line

SHOULD THE TUBES ON A CENTRAL LINE BE CLAMPED OFF?

No. Persistently used clamps may cause erosion in the tubing.

IF THE TUBE BECOMES DISCONNECTED BELOW THE CLAMPS ON A HICKMAN OR BROVIAC CATHETER, WHAT SHOULD I DO?

Clamp the tube in the center or bend the tubing over and use a Foley C clamp or needle cap, or hold the tubing together and prevent an air embolism.

WHAT SHOULD I DO IF THE PATIENT HAS NO DRESSING OVER THE CENTRAL LINE?

Unless the line is an implantable port, cover the site with a sterile dressing until the site can be properly cleansed and redressed, using the facility procedure for applying a central line dressing.

DO I NEED TO WORRY ABOUT WHICH PORT IS FOR DRAWING BLOOD AND WHICH PORT(S) IS FOR INFUSING FLUIDS?

Not in the triage area. If the patient has reported one of the ports as nonfunctioning, the nonfunctioning port should be flagged with silk tape to indicate that it needs particularly careful evaluation.

---

comfortable with the devices, or they should triage the patient as emergent if no peers are available for consultation. Care should be taken in dealing with central lines to not break sterile barriers without using sterile technique, and the triage nurse and care providers should not use scissors or other sharp items near the line, even when discontinuing the dressing (Freedman and Bosserman, 1993).

Chest Tubes

Most community-based patients require chest tubes for draining pleural fluid, usually because of buildup of pleural fluid in patients who have cancer with metastatic involvement or in patients with primary lung cancer.

Patients with chest tubes seek care in EDs most commonly because the collection chamber attached to the chest tubes is full or because there is a difficulty with chest tube patency or fluid drainage. The triage of the patient depends on the specific reason for seeking care and whether the patient has a complaint that involves chest discomfort or respiratory discomfort or distress. As mentioned earlier, patients with invasive equipment sometimes seek care for reasons unrelated to the function of their medical equipment. Patients with chest tubes should have immediate attention by the triage nurse, since they are at high risk for thoracic problems. The only time patients with chest tubes are not considered ''urgent'' is when they clearly indicate that they are there for a change of the fluid collection system and there is still sufficient collection space in the fluid collection chamber for safe waiting.

Triage questions that should be asked of the patient with chest tubes are directed by the chief complaint and physical appearance of the patient. Patients with chest or respiratory discomfort or distress should be asked the triage questions identified in Chapter 7 (Box 7–3). If the patient is not in distress or discomfort but has a nonimmediate concern related to the function, nature, or collection of plural fluid drainage, questions specific to the equipment and reason for chest tube placement should be asked. Patients should be asked why the chest tubes were placed, when they were placed, how the procedure was tolerated, how long the patients have been home with the chest tubes, and how the patients are being monitored and cared for. Patients should also be queried about the most recent visit to their primary care provider and the results of the visit. Specific questions regarding the amount of pleural fluid output over a specific period of time should follow, as well as a request for the description of the character of the fluid. Patients should be asked how they are feeling in general and how they are replacing the fluid lost through the chest tube (e.g., diet, intravenous therapy, or tube feeding). General triage questions that should be asked of patients with chest tubes are listed in Box 11–9.

Advance directives must be explored with patients or family members of patients with primary lung cancer or metastatic lung involvement who are in distress or likely to require

BOX 11-9 | **Triage Questions for the Patient With Chest Tubes**

What is the reason you are seeking care?

Do you have chest discomfort? (If the answer is yes, immediately do a symptom analysis of the chest discomfort.)

Are you having new or increased difficulty breathing or feeling that you are not getting enough air? (If the answer is yes, immediately do a symptom analysis of respiratory difficulty.)

Why do you have chest tube(s)? When was chest tube insertion performed?

How have you been managing at home with the chest tubes? (Who takes care of monitoring the drainage and function of the equipment?)

When was your most recent visit to your primary care provider? What was the result of the visit?

What is the amount of pleural fluid you have noticed? Over what period of time?

Has there been a sudden increase or decrease in the drainage?

Please describe the character of the fluid.

How are you replacing the fluid lost through the chest tube?

If patient is an oncology patient or terminal with other pathology, the triage nurse may ask about a living will if the patient is comfortable and department policies do not contraindicate an inquiry of this nature in triage.

---

aggressive acute care and with patients who are mortally ill. Patients often have documents that request the withholding of aggressive intervention in the case of cardiopulmonary arrest, but in the rush to go to the hospital the documents are not brought to the facility. If inquiries about advance directives are made at once, it is sometimes possible for family, friends, or care providers to arrange for the necessary documents to be made available to hospital personnel. This may expedite the legal withholding of aggressive medical interventions, which would increase the suffering of a patient with a terminal condition whose wishes are not consistent with aggressive medical care. Conversely, if a patient has a desire for full resuscitation, this may also be clearly indicated on the chart so that value judgments based on the patient's diagnosis do not cloud the obligations of acute-care providers.

Physical assessment of the patient with chest tubes. The chest tube insertion site should be examined for dressing integrity if easily accessible. If the chest tube site is not easily accessible to the triage nurse and the environment does not enable the patient to have privacy, the patient can be asked to describe the appearance of the dressing. The dressing should be occlusive and without fresh drainage. If the patient has fresh drainage, the nurse should record the characteristics of the drainage and ask the patient when she/he first observed the drainage. If the patient has drainage on the dressing that raises suspicion of infection, the patient should be asked about symptoms of sepsis (e.g., fever and chills) at home. The skin surrounding the chest tube insertion site should be inspected for signs of inflammation and palpated for crepitation. Patients with respiratory difficulty should have their oxygen saturation measured by pulse oximetry, and auscultation for breath sounds should be performed to assess for bilateral breath sounds or, in the patient with a lobectomy, to determine whether breath sounds are present over all existing lung fields. Even if the chest tube has been placed to maintain inflation of the lung, pulmonary perforation, although rare, may be a complication of chest tube insertion (Resnick, 1993). Complications associated with chest tube insertion are listed in Box 11–10.

The patient's trachea should be observed for deviation, which may indicate pneumothorax or hemothorax. Patients with critical physical assessment findings should, of course, be triaged for immediate care. The chest tubes should be assessed for patency, and an observation made for secure connections to the collection system. Functioning of all chambers should appear to be consistent with manufacturer's specifications. If the chest tubes do not appear to be draining, the nurse should consider the general configuration of the patient. Morbid obesity can cause collapse and kinking of chest tubes in the subcutaneous and fatty tissue (Iberti and Stern, 1992). The chest drainage unit should be below the level of the patient's chest to permit gravity drainage flow (*Nursing*, 1993). Fluid draining into a fluid collection chamber should be observed for amount, color, and char-

| BOX 11–10 | **Complications Associated With Chest Tube Insertion** |

- Lung perforation
- Empyema
- Residual pneumothorax
- Placement of the tube in the chest wall
- Diaphragmatic perforation
- Perforation of intraabdominal organs (spleen, liver, or stomach)
- Unilateral pulmonary edema
- Bronchopleural fistula
- Hemothorax
- Cardiogenic shock
- Horner's syndrome

| BOX 11–11 | **Physical Assessment in Triage of the Patient With Chest Tubes** |

- Inspect and palpate the trachea for deviation (if helpful, place one finger above the suprasternal notch to verify midline placement by light palpation of the trachea).
- Observe the patient for signs of respiratory distress (bulging and retraction of intercostal space, use of accessory muscles, tachypnea or bradypnea, cyanosis or pallor, and general signs of increased respiratory effort).*
- Observe the chest tube insertion site for presence of an occlusive dressing.
- Inspect the condition of the dressing, and record the nature and amount of any discharge on the dressing.
- Inspect the taping of the chest tube to be sure it is secure.
- Palpate tissue surrounding chest tube insertion site for crepitation.
- Auscultate the patient's lung fields for breath sounds with particular attention to the presence of diminished or absent breath sounds. (Consider patient's unique anatomy if lobectomy has been performed.)
- Inspect the chest tubes for patency, and record the color, character, and amount of pleural fluid.
- Assess oxygen saturation by pulse oximetry if available.

*Determine whether the patient's signs and symptoms are chronic or new by asking care provider or significant other if necessary.

acteristics, and documentation made about this finding. If the fluid has an enteric character, delayed perforation of the esophagus or stomach should be suspected (Shapira et al., 1993) and the patient should be triaged as emergent for ED care. This complication is more common with a posteriorly placed chest tube. When the patient has persistent or excessive bloody drainage in the chest tubes an immediate investigation into the cause is necessary, since this complication has been linked to injury to intercostal or pulmonary vessels or to a leaking aortic aneurysm (Muthuswamy et al., 1993).

Patients suspected of having hemodynamic instability may need auscultation of the apical pulse if verification of normal cardiac rate and rhythm is necessary; attention to the patient with tachycardia or bradycardia should be thorough. Furthermore, orthostatic vital signs should be assessed if patients complain of dizziness or if the nurse intuitively feels that this assessment measure is warranted. An overview of physical assessment measures that should be performed in triage of patients with chest tubes is provided in Box 11–11. Indications that immediate care might be necessary for patients with chest tubes are listed in Box 11–12.

BOX 11–12	**Indications for Possible Emergent Triage Designation in Patients With Chest Tubes**

- Acute respiratory distress or chest discomfort
- Oxygen saturation <90% on pulse oximetry
- Signs of pneumothorax or hemothorax (tracheal deviation; unequal, diminished, or absent breath sounds over any lung field, presence of palpable crepitation, and the like)
- Obvious sepsis (temperature >101° F oral and so forth)
- Sudden or excessive increase in pleural fluid output beyond expected amount, as indicated by patient or primary care provider
- Change from previously clear pleural fluid drainage to bloody drainage
- Completely full pleural fluid collection chamber
- Signs of hemodynamic instability (tachycardia, hypotension, and orthostatic vital sign changes)

Patients who seek emergency care for a change of the fluid collection equipment attached to their chest tube(s) may be safely considered ''nonurgent'' if their triage history and physical assessment indicate that they are otherwise in stable condition. The primary health care provider should be contacted to determine whether the patient may safely be triaged to clinic or office for care or should be seen within the ED. Patients with concerns regarding chest tubes or with chief complaints related to the thorax are triaged as urgent or emergent in the absence of level-4 criteria and if they are physically unable to tolerate a longer waiting period.

Urinary Tract Catheters

Patients with indwelling urinary tract catheters or patients who use other catheter procedures or devices at home may seek emergency care for a variety of reasons. If during the triage interview and assessment the nurse thinks that the patient is likely to have a catheter inserted or removed, she/he should ask about the patient's general medical history. Patients with cardiac disease that may predispose them to bacterial endocarditis should be given prophylactic antibiotics prior to the insertion or removal of a catheter (Gillenwater, 1991). If the patient is in great discomfort, the triage nurse should communicate the medical history as soon as possible to the primary physician or the ED physician.

All patients with catheters should be questioned about the reasons for catheter use, the type of catheter used, signs of local inflammation or infection related to the catheter itself, history of catheter-related difficulties, contact with primary health care provider, and treatments and medications used at home to relieve symptoms related to the chief complaint (Box 11–13). Since indwelling catheters are made of silicon-coated latex, the patient should be asked about known allergies to latex. This is particularly crucial in children with spina bifida, who are the patients most commonly diagnosed with latex hypersensitivity (Schneck and Bellinger, 1993). Symptoms of latex allergy may be as minor as cough and as severe as bronchospasm and anaphylaxis (Ellsworth et al., 1993).

The mode of catheter care should be determined. All patients should be using proper hand washing before handling or

BOX 11–13	**Triage Questions for Patients Using Urinary Tract Catheter Devices**

- Do you have abdominal discomfort? (If yes, perform a symptom analysis of the patient's abdominal discomfort.)
- How long have you been using this device? What is the reason for use?
- What type of catheter do you use (brand name, size, and type)?
- What hygiene measures do you use to reduce your risk of catheter-related infections?
- Have you noticed signs of local inflammation or infection related to the catheter itself?
- Do you have a history of catheter-related difficulties?
- How and exactly where on your leg or body do you secure the catheter (if indwelling)?
- Have you used treatments or medications at home to relieve symptoms related to the problem you have identified today?
- Are you allergic to latex?
- Have you noticed a change in the color, odor, amount, or characteristics of your urine? If so, please describe.
- If the catheter is indwelling, how often do you empty your drainage device?

STRAIGHT CATHETERS

How do you store your catheter?
How frequently do you exchange your catheter for a new one?
How often do you catheterize yourself or are you catheterized?

EXTERNAL CATHETER DEVICES

How often do you clean under the catheter?
How do you clean the area of skin under the catheter? (What do you use as a cleaning agent?)
How is the catheter held in place?

---

caring for the catheter, observing their urine for color and amount, and taking care to maintain a closed system through proper handling of the catheter and collection system (Burden, 1993). The drainage collection container should be emptied at least every 8 hours. This procedure should be confirmed with the patient. If the patient has a leg bag, it should be emptied at least every 2 hours during the day (Brechtelsbauer, 1992).

Patients who use straight-catheter equipment and procedures should be asked about their procedure for cleaning the catheter, storage of the catheter, how frequently the catheter is exchanged for a new one, and the frequency with which they catheterize themselves or are catheterized. Children who self-catheterize are at higher risk of bacteriuria, since they may be less rigorous in maintaining proper cleanliness during catheterization and catheter care (Gillenwater, 1991). Straight catheterization of infants with size 5 or 8 French feeding tubes has been associated with obstruction that is due to excessive tube insertion in the bladder, which causes the tubing to knot, thereby impeding removal (Foster et al., 1992). For infants who arrive at the ED with a report of straight-catheter difficulties, the type of tubing used and method of insertion should be determined. In assessing the patient's catheter system, the nurse should confirm that the drainage bag is below the level of the bladder.

The most common problem associated with routine catheter use, straight or indwelling, is infection. Patients with a chief complaint of abdominal pain or suspected urinary tract infection should be evaluated using a symptom analysis for this problem (see Chapter 5, Box 5–1). The risk of infection is highest in elderly or disabled patients, in patients with urologic abnormalities, and in pregnant women (Gillenwater, 1991). Virtually all patients with indwelling catheters at some time have a urinary tract infection; sometimes the bacteria are resistant to a number of antibiotics. Therefore it is helpful for the triage nurse not only to interview the patient about her/his symptoms but also to reinforce use of measures that help prevent infections.

Patients with external catheter devices should be asked about the type and frequency of care for skin under the catheter and how the catheter is held in place. Men with condom catheters sometimes have obstruction of urinary flow and resultant urinary tract infections when occlusive devices are used too rigorously or inappropriately to keep the catheter in place. Infections may occur in patients who have external catheter devices when the patient is uncooperative or confused and tends to pull on the catheter (Gillenwater, 1991).

It is not practical to observe the placement of the catheter at triage unless the patient is an infant or the triage or assessment area is completely private. Whatever part of indwelling catheter equipment is available for inspection should be observed for tube condition and patency, and the fluid collection chamber should be observed for color, amount, and characteristics of urine. Collection of a urine sample should not be performed in the triage area, since the sterile procedure that should be used is more successfully carried out within the ED.

Patients seeking emergency care for obstruction of a catheter or for difficulty in using a straight catheter caused by a mechanical obstruction should be asked about the amount of urine they have had, when they noticed the decrease or impossibility of output, and the presence of abdominal discomfort. Patients who have not voided in 12 or more hours or who are in acute discomfort should be seen immediately and, when physician ordered, catheterized as soon as possible in the ED.

REFERENCES

Brechtelsbauer D: Care with an indwelling urinary catheter: tips for avoiding problems in independent and institutionalized patients, *Postgrad Med* 92(1):127, 1992.

Burden N: *Ambulatory surgical nursing,* Philadelphia, 1993, WB Saunders.

Camp-Sorrell O: Implantable ports: everything you always wanted to know, *J Intraven Nurs* 15(5):262, 1992.

Cowan C: Antibiotic lock technique, *J Intraven Nurs* 15(5):283, 1993.

Ellsworth P et al: Evaluation and risk factors of latex allergy in spina bifida patients: is it preventable? *J Urol* 150(pt 2):691, 1993.

Ena J et al: Cross-sectional epidemiology of phlebitis and catheter-related infections, *Infect Control Hosp Epidemiol* 13(1):15, 1992.

Foster H, Ritchey M, Bloom D: Adventitious knots in urethral catheters: report of 5 cases, *J Urol* 148(5):1496, 1992.

Freedman S, Bosserman G: Tunneled catheters: technologic advances and nursing care issues, *Nurs Clin North Am* 28(4):851, 1993.

Gillenwater J: *Adult and pediatric urology,* ed 2, St Louis, 1991, Mosby.

Groeger J et al: Infectious morbidity associated with long-term use of venous access devices in patients with cancer, *Ann Intern Med* 119(12):1168, 1993.

Iberti T, Stern P: Chest tube thoracostomy, *Crit Care Clin* 8(4):879, 1992.

Kitt S, Kaiser J: *Emergency nursing: a physiologic and clinical perspective,* Philadelphia, 1990, WB Saunders.

Managing chest drainage problems, *Nursing* 23(8):32J, 1993.

Muthuswamy P et al: Recurrent massive bleeding from an intercostal artery aneurysm through an empyema chest tube, *Chest* 104(2):637, 1993.

Orr ME: Issues in the management of percutaneous central venous catheters: single and multiple lumens, *Nurs Clin North Am* 28(4):911, 1993.

Orr M, Ryder M: Vascular access devices: perspectives on designs, complications, and management, *Nutr Clin Pract* 8(4):145, 1993.

Pauley S et al: Catheter-related colonization associated with percutaneous inserted central catheters, *J Intraven Nurs* 16(1):51, 1993.

Potter P, Perry A: *Clinical nursing skills and techniques,* ed 3, St Louis, 1994, Mosby.

Puel V et al: Superior vena cava thrombosis related to catheter malposition in cancer chemotherapy given through implanted ports, *Cancer* 72(7):2248, 1993.

Raad I et al: The relationship between the thrombotic and infectious complications of central venous catheters, *JAMA* 271(13):1014, 1994.

Resnick D: Delayed pulmonary perforation: a rare complication of tube thoracostomy, *Chest* 103(1):311, 1993.

Sariego J et al: Major long-term complications in 1,422 permanent venous access devices, *Am J Surg* 165(2):249, 1993.

Schneck F, Bellinger M: The ''innocent'' cough or sneeze: a harbinger of serious latex allergy in children during bladder stimulation and urodynamic testing, *J Urol* 150(pt 2):687, 1993.

Shapira O et al: Delayed perforation of the esophagus by a closed thoracostomy tube, *Chest* 104(6):1897, 1993.

RECOMMENDED READING

Birdwell G, Yeager R, Whitsett T: Pseudotumor cerebri: a complication of catheter-induced subclavian vein thrombosis, *Arch Intern Med* 154(7):808, 1994.

Gullo S: Implanted ports: technologic advances and nursing care issues, *Nurs Clin North Am* 28(4):859, 1993.

Manheimer F, Aranda C, Smith R: Necrotizing pneumonitis caused by 5-fluorouracil infusion: a complication of a Hickman catheter, *Cancer* 70(2):554, 1992.

Mergaert S: S.T.O.P. and assess chest tubes the easy way, *Nursing* 24(2):52, 1992.

Raad I et al: Low infection rate and long durability of nontunneled Silastic catheters: a safe and cost-effective alternative for long-term venous access, *Arch Intern Med* 153(15):1791, 1993.

Tanagh O, Emil A, McAninch J: *Smith's general urology,* ed 13, 1992, Appleton & Lange.

Winkler T et al: Unusual cause of hemoptysis: Hickman-induced cavabronchial fistula, *Chest* 102(4):1285, 1993.

12 | Psychiatric Crises

With the exception of the trauma patient, no patient has the ability to influence the milieu of the emergency department (ED) as dramatically as the psychiatric patient. Because psychiatric patients can be extremely unpredictable, frightening, and frustrating to care for, nurses respond with varying degrees of trepidation and avoidance. In providing a number of these individuals with comforting reassurance, safety, and compassion there is an opportunity to experience unforgettable professional satisfaction and, if not the most satisfying experience in your nursing career, perhaps the most unique.

Patients who need psychiatric interventions can range from a muscular, 6-foot-tall man who has become psychotic and must be restrained to prevent him from running about the ED, to a parent who is overwhelmingly distraught as her child clings to life, to a homeless man who is suicidal because his best friend for 13 years, "a mutt of a dog," had died.

Having the opportunity to provide a grief-stricken parent with the support and comfort she desperately needs or arranging for a trip to the pound to pick up another stray mutt can give an ED nurse a tremendous amount of gratification.

THE PSYCHIATRIC PATIENT

Disorders in individuals who require emergent psychiatric care may be classified into six broad categories (Box 12–1). This categorization, however, does not imply that patients remain exclusive to one category. Psychiatric patients frequently arrive at triage with several signs and symptoms that could be classified into several categories simultaneously, for example, an elderly patient with a psychotic depression, a suicidal alcoholic, or a schizophrenic in crisis after being thrown out of his parents' home because of substance abuse.

BOX 12–1	**Categories of Disorders in Psychiatric Patients**

THOUGHT DISORDER, TYPICALLY PSYCHOSIS

Schizophrenia

MOOD DISORDERS

Major depression and mania

PERSONALITY DISORDERS

Borderline, antisocial, histrionic, multipersonality

SITUATIONAL CRISIS

An insufficient ability to cope after an overwhelming event; patients may include an individual who has had a sudden death of family member, a developmentally disabled adolescent whose behavior is out of control, or a victim of rape

PSYCHOLOGIC DISTURBANCES WITH BIOLOGIC OR MEDICAL ORIGINS

Organic brain syndrome, Alzheimer's disease, multiinfarct dementia, AIDS, chronic pain, intracranial tumors, Huntington's disease, alcohol and drug intoxication, and other disturbances

OTHER

Diagnoses that are not clearly classified into the other categories, such as obsessive-compulsive disorder, posttraumatic stress disorder

ASSESSMENT

The ability to rapidly and accurately assess the psychiatric patient depends on the complexity of the patient's condition and the skill of the nurse. A complete, thorough assessment includes a mental status examination (MSE), a history of the patient's current and past medications and treatment, and a social, work, and family history.

For the triage nurse the most practical approach would be to complete an MSE and medication history. The MSE might be considered an elaboration of "people-watching" at the shopping mall or the airport. Much can be learned about a person by

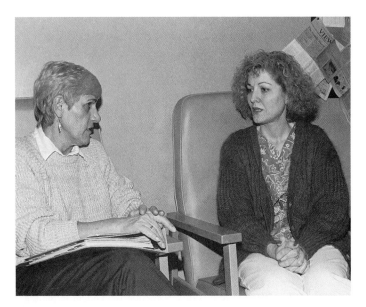

Fig. 12–1 The mental health interview takes place in a comfortable setting.

methodic observation. How individuals respond to the nurse's introduction and the information they provide in a brief interview usually verify the first impression of an experienced clinician. It is important to remember that the MSE is not just an assessment but is also an intervention. By calmly and supportively asking patients about themselves, it is possible to make the patient already begin to feel a sense of relief (Fig. 12–1).

The complete MSE includes the components listed in Box 12–2.

An excellent way to practice doing the MSE is simply to "people watch" and methodically observe such characteristics as the activity and affect of people, perhaps of the hallucinating street person, a "stressed-out" mother in the grocery store who is verbally abusing her child, or a depressed teenager on the bus. If you are in an outgoing mood, muster the courage to attempt to verify your observations. The most useful approach in verifying your "hunch" is to be neither assumptive nor judg-

BOX 12–2	Psychiatric Mental Status Examination

APPEARANCE

How does the patient look? Is she/he well groomed? How is she/he dressed?

ACTIVITY

How does the patient move about or walk? Is there psychomotor agitation or retardation? Pacing? Odd, inexplicable movements (i.e., *posturing*)? Assess for notable gestures, tics, or involuntary movements.

AFFECT

Affect is the nurse's assessment of the patient's mood. Does the patient look angry, depressed, elated, or suspicious? Is the patient's expression appropriate to the actions or words of the patient? Does the expression quickly change (i.e., *affect is labile*)? Is it difficult to determine whether the patient is feeling anything (i.e., is there a *flat* or *blunted affect*)?

EYE CONTACT

Is eye contact a fixed stare? Are the eyes darting about? Does the patient avoid eye contact? Are the patient's eyes even open?

SPEECH

What is the rate of speech? Is it slow or rapid? Is the patient mute? What is the volume of speech? Is the speech clear or slurred? Are there strange patterns or words in what the patient is saying or how she/he is saying it?

MOOD

Mood is the feeling that the patient states he/she has.

THOUGHT

There are two parts to this assessment: content and process. The severity of the patient's illness is often identifiable by what the patient is thinking and how the patient is able to organize and communicate those thoughts.

> *Content.* Is the patient delusional (i.e., does the patient have a *fixed, false belief, despite obvious evidence to the contrary*)? Delusions may be religiously based, somatic, or persecutory.

| BOX 12–2 | Psychiatric Mental Status Examination—cont'd |

Is the patient actively hallucinating (i.e., having a *false perception with no real stimulus*), either auditory, visual, olfactory, or tactile? Is the patient illusional (i.e., having *a false perception of a real stimulus,* such as believing it is God who is speaking through the intercom)? Is the patient telling you that everything she/he sees or encounters is somehow connected or related to the patient personally (i.e., having *ideas of reference*)? Is the patient suicidal? Homicidal?

Process. Are the patient's thoughts organized? Does the patient rapidly switch from one slightly connected thought to another (i.e., having *flight of ideas*)? Are the thoughts totally disorganized? Does the patient go into excessive detail before reaching a conclusion (i.e., does the patient have *circumstantial* thoughts)? Does the patient suddenly stop in the middle of a sentence (i.e., is there *thought blocking*)?

ORIENTATION

Assess orientation to person, place, and time. A patient should be able to tell the nurse the patient's name and age; what city the patient is in; the day of the week, the month, and the season of the year.

MEMORY

Short-term and long-term memory should be assessed. Ask the patient what she/he had for breakfast. Where does the patient live? Who is the president of the United States?

mental; instead, be reflective. A short supportive sentence or two, even from a complete stranger, can make a difference in the day of someone who may be depressed, under stress, or anxious.

ASSESSMENT OF MEDICATION

As in all patients, it is important to assess the patient's current and past medication regimens. What medication is the patient

---

| BOX 12–3 | Medication Assessment Caution |

If a patient's mental status is in question, be alert in listening to
what the patient tells you regarding the medication history. If a
patient's mental status is clearly compromised, other sources of
information should be sought. Is there a family member or friend
present? Has the patient been hospitalized there previously, and
is an old chart available? If the patient is receiving follow-up
care from a community mental health center, there is usually a
mental health therapist who is on call and should be contacted.
Often these professionals not only provide useful medication
history but also are familiar with rehospitalization patterns for a
particular individual or other pertinent information. Recidivism
for patients with schizophrenia because of noncompliance with
medication regimens is quite common, and a careful evaluation
of a psychotic patient's medication history facilitates rapid
treatment and release of the patient.

---

currently taking? Be sure to include the dose and dosage. Does
the patient take any medication on an "as needed" basis? What
medications have been tried in the past? Depending on the patient's mental status, it may not be possible to obtain an accurate
medication history (Box 12–3).

It is good policy, for the safety of the patient and others,
to ask the patient to allow you to keep the medications that are
in the patient's possession until the patient can be further evaluated by the mental health staff.

SPECIFIC ASSESSMENT FINDINGS AND INTERVENTIONS

There are dozens of diagnoses for which the psychiatric patient
enters the ED. Several of the most common diagnoses are discussed in detail in this chapter. To discuss assessment and management of the psychiatric patient completely, an entire book
would have to be written. Please refer to the references at the
end of this chapter for further resources.

Thought Disorders: Schizophrenia

According to the *Diagnostic and Statistical Manual of Mental Disorders, Fourth Edition* (1994), someone may be diagnosed as having schizophrenia only if the person has psychotic symptoms, a decrease in normal level of functioning in areas such as personal life, work, and social life over a period of at least 6 months, and an onset that occurs before the age of 45 years.

Assessment and interventions

Appearance. The patient is unkempt, sometimes has odd matching of clothes, and is malodorous. If the patient is, indeed, very dirty and smells bad, set the expectation that the patient will be showered shortly by stating, ''It looks like you haven't been able to get to a shower lately. You can look forward to the staff showing you where to bathe.''

Activity. For the psychotic patient who is on a regimen of antipsychotic (i.e., neuroleptic) medications, activity is the most difficult area for the practitioner to assess. Agitation or bizarre movements may be caused by disturbing hallucinations or may be side effects of the medication the patient is currently taking. If the patient is currently taking neuroleptic medications (especially high-potency, low-dosage medications) and is clearly agitated or is posturing, the following extrapyramidal side effects should be assessed.

Akathisia is an inability to sit still. It is important to clarify why the patient cannot sit down. Observe the patient when he/she is sitting. Is the patient rubbing the legs or bouncing them up and down on the toes?

Bradykinesia is the opposite of akathisia. The patient may be mistaken for someone who is quite depressed. In more serious forms, the patient may appear catatonic.

Dystonia is a severe, uncomfortable cramp that most often affects the head or neck muscles.

Treatment for the three side effects just mentioned is simple and often provides quick relief. Typically, either diphenhydramine (Benadryl) 50 mg or benztropine mesylate (Cogentin) 1 to 2 mg is given intra-

muscularly. If the symptoms are not relieved, lorazepam (Ativan) or a similar benzodiazepine will be
tried.

A disturbing chronic side effect of neuroleptic medication is *tardive dyskinesia*. Tardive dyskinesia is
usually found in older adults who have been on a regimen of neuroleptics for a prolonged period. It is dis-
figuring and in severe forms almost disabling. Signs
of tardive dyskinesia are frequent eye blinking, lip
smacking or puckering, chewing movements, and constant sticking out of the tongue. There is no effective
treatment.

If the patient's behavior is related to hallucinations,
set clear, firm limits in a nonthreatening way on what
is appropriate behavior for a public area. (For example, make a statement such as, ''Your behavior of
flapping your arms like a bird and howling is frightening the other patients here and will not be tolerated.
Please remain seated. Someone will be with you in 20
[or the like] minutes.'') If verbal limits are not followed, remove the patient from the area and medicate
the patient as soon as possible.

Affect. Patient's mood is assessed to be flat, inappropriate,
and fearful.

Eye contact. A patient who is actively hallucinating appears distracted and does not make much eye contact.
Paranoid individuals occasionally wear sunglasses.

Speech. Speech is rambling and incoherent. Hallucinating
patients stop talking because of an interruption by the
voices they hear. Paranoid patients may remain mute.
Sometimes totally unrelated words are strung together in
a sentence (*word salad*), or the patient invents words that
have meaning only to the patient (*neologisms*).

Mood. The patient's mood varies and may quickly change.

Thought. Delusions may be present. If present, they are
usually grandiose or paranoid and often involve God, the
Federal Bureau of Investigation (FBI), or the Central Intelligence Agency (CIA). Auditory hallucinations are the
most common type. Ask the patient what the voices are

saying. Command hallucinations (voices instructing the patient to do or say certain things) that are destructive are a "red flag" for the nurse. The patient should receive immediate attention and one-to-one supervision until the condition is stabilized. Other voices may be arguing, commenting, or laughing and are less of a threat to the patient, to others, or to the environment. Psychotic individuals may have circumstantial thinking or thought blocking.

Avoid whispering or laughing in front of the paranoid patient, since this may escalate the paranoia. Tactfully express doubt about the reality of the voices, and assist the patient with thought dismissal by making statements such as, "I cannot hear the voices in your head. Tell them to go away and leave you alone."

Orientation. Patients are usually oriented unless extremely paranoid and mute. Reorient the patient as needed.

Memory. The patient's memory is intact.

Other interventions

Consider hydration and nutrition in the grossly disorganized patient. If possible, offer the patient a drink and snack. Monitor the patient's behavior to determine whether the patient knows what to do with the drink and food.

Avoid trying to comfort patient by gentle touching on the arm or shoulder.

Be in control. As bizarre and startling as a patient's behavior might be, do not let the patient see any apprehension from you.

Management of the violent patient is discussed later in this chapter.

Mood Disorders: Major Depression With Suicidal Ideation

Feeling depressed or sad is different from being classified as having major depression. The diagnosis of major depression requires the presence, for 2 weeks or more, of several signs or

---

BOX 12–4	**Individuals at Greatest Risk for Suicide Attempts**

- Unmarried older men
- White persons
- Unemployed persons
- Individuals in poor physical health
- Persons living alone
- Patients dealing with an anniversary of a death or loss
- Individuals facing a sudden, dramatic change in life

---

symptoms such as increased irritability, sleep disturbance (either much more or less sleep than usual), weight gain or loss, loss of energy, and decreased concentration. Suicidal ideation is the presence of thoughts of harming oneself (Box 12–4).

Assessment

Appearance. Careless, unkempt appearance is common.

Activity. Psychomotor retardation, slouched posture, or agitation is present.

Affect. Depressed, flat affect is evident.

Eye contact. Eye contact is poor, and the patient may be tearful.

Speech. Patient's speech is soft and slow.

Mood. Hopeless, helpless, depressed, angry, or irritable.

Thought. Inquiring about someone's thoughts of harming herself/himself does not increase the risk to the suicidal individual. Ask the patient what the plans are. Is the plan lethal? The more serious the plan (cutting the throat is more serious than swallowing 10 Tylenol tablets), the greater the risk. Is the plan available to the patient? The greater the availability, the greater the risk. If the means to harm self (or others) is immediately available to the patient, for example, the patient is carrying a gun, remove it at once.

A depressed, suicidal patient may be ambivalent about being admitted into the hospital, and questions regarding hallucinations may insult the patient and negatively influence the patient's desire to seek admission. An explanatory preamble to assessment for the presence of hallucinations, such as the following, typically suffices: *"When individuals are in crisis and extremely distraught, their minds sometimes play tricks on them. Have you heard any voices in your head but didn't know where they came from?"* Hallucinations are uncommon and, if present, are usually in elderly patients who have been withdrawn and isolated.

Orientation. The patient is oriented.

Memory. The patient's memory is intact.

Interventions

If the patient cannot be treated immediately, *contract a verbal or written "no harm" agreement* while the patient is waiting. It should be specific, for example, "I, John Doe, promise not to harm myself while in the hospital the next 4 hours. If I have very impulsive feelings to do so, I will seek out staff for assistance." If the patient is not able to make such a contract or is not releasable, one-to-one observations should be initiated.

Do not attempt to establish rapport by "keeping a secret." If a patient offers information with stipulations, inform the patient that you are part of a team that will care for the patient and that any relevant information the patient shares with you must be passed along to the team. Usually the individual divulges the information.

Avoid saying, "I know how you feel." Instead, recognize the patient's feelings by stating, "I can see that you are extremely upset about this. We will provide you with a safe environment and do our best to help you overcome this crisis."

Personality Disorders: Borderline Personality

Patients with a personality disorder often represent the most difficult type of individual for the triage nurse to care for. Many of these patients have deficient, harmful methods of coping with personal stress and often come to the ED with the expectation that the staff will resolve their current crisis for them.

Twelve personality disorders are listed in the DSM-IV.

Several of these disorders are relatively common in the ED, but the borderline and antisocial personality disorders represent the greatest challenge in acute health care management. Because these patients are quite unpredictable, there are no "common" findings in the MSE. The borderline personality disorder can be an extremely complicated condition to manage. The diagnostic criteria for the borderline personality disorder are given in Box 12–5, and in reviewing these criteria the nurse may develop an appreciation for the complexity these patients present to the hospital staff.

Interventions

Establish "no-harm" contracts, and *initiate close observation* of the patient. The potential for self-harm is high in individuals with personality disorders, and it is not unusual for them to carry out such acts near or even in the presence of health care providers.

Set limits on rude, "acting out" behavior.

BOX 12–5	**Borderline Personality Disorder**

The DSM-IV requires at least five of the following eight criteria, for the diagnosis of borderline personality disorder:

1. Impulsivity or unpredictability in at least two areas that are potentially self-damaging, such as spending, sex, gambling, substance abuse, or physically self-damaging acts
2. A long-term pattern of intense but unstable interpersonal relationships as evidence by marked shifts in feelings, idealization, devaluation, or manipulation
3. Inappropriate, intense anger
4. Identity disturbance manifested by uncertainty about several issues such as self-image, gender identity, career choice, values, or loyalties
5. Affective instability
6. Intolerance of being alone
7. Physically self-damaging acts such as suicidal gestures or self-mutilation.
8. Chronic feelings of emptiness or boredom

Many patients with borderline personality disorder are masters at manipulation. With a patient who has chronic complaints of crisis, the staff avoids being split (i.e., taking sides on how to treat the patient) by *establishing a care plan*. An effective care plan should include the following:

Criteria for admission. Will the patient contract no harm? Does the patient agree to a short stay (generally 5 days or less)? Does the patient have a referral from the outpatient therapist?

Appropriate ED interventions. For example, the care plan may specify that staff will spend 10 minutes with the patient every hour until the patient is transferred to the unit or that only certain medications will be administered by the ED staff.

A *careful self-assessment* of the nurse's feelings toward these patients is an important intervention. Recognition of the challenges and discussion among staff foster an attitude that facilitates treatment of these patients.

Management of the violent patient is discussed later in this chapter.

Situational Crisis: Anxiety Disorder

The panic-stricken or overly anxious patient is fairly common in the ED. As with the patient who has borderline personality disorder, patients with anxiety may become well known to the ED staff. For first-time patients, however, differentiating a medical illness from a psychophysiologic disorder can be challenging. A brief medical and family history and an MSE can provide enough accurate data to determine the origin of the anxiety or panic.

Assessment and interventions

Appearance. Grooming is typically not a problem.

Activity. Patient may be restless or sweating; a fine tremor may be present; hyperventilation may be present. The patient may be tremulous.

Have the patient sit down, close both eyes, and concentrate on slowed breathing. Talk to the patient in a quiet, calm, reassuring voice. If the patient is unable to slow the breathing down, ask the patient to breathe into a paper bag. If this intervention is unsuccessful, the patient may try lying face down on the floor with arms extended above the head. Benzodiazepines are beneficial for patients who cannot recover from a panic attack.

Affect. Fretful, apprehensive affect is evident.

Eye contact. Good eye contact is made. The patient's eyes may be darting.

Speech. Rapid, short sentences result from hyperventilation or tightness in the chest. Ask the patient to try and slow the speech down.

Mood. The patient may feel afraid.

Thought. Feelings of impending doom and helplessness are common. Patient may fear becoming insane or violent and may have negative hallucinations or delusions. Thought process is usually organized, articulate. If the panic attacks have been fairly common, the patient is at risk for suicidal ideation and should be assessed once the anxiety begins to diminish. It is therapeutic to have the patient express fears and, at the same time, to directly explain the patient's symptoms and unrealistic fears. If possible, decrease the patient's environmental stimuli. Reassure the patient that she/he will not lose control of her/his behavior or sanity.

Orientation. Patient is oriented to person, place, and time.

Memory. Patient's memory is intact.

Psychologic Disturbances Resulting From Biologic or Medical Causes: Alcoholism

Along with tobacco, alcohol is one of the most significant contributors to poor health, and like anxiety disorders, alcohol-related problems are common in the ED. The clinical effects of alcohol are present when the blood alcohol level is greater than 100 mg. Stupor is typically seen at levels around 300 mg; levels of 400 to 600 mg result in unconsciousness; and levels above 600 mg can result in death, although individuals usually pass out before such high blood alcohol levels are reached.

Assessment

Mental status examination. The patient is almost always accompanied by a police officer, family member, or friend. The patient looks disheveled and dirty. The patient either is greatly assisted while walking or has an uncoordinated gait. There is the potential for combativeness. The affect can range from irritable and angry to elated or ''lost.'' Eye contact is difficult to maintain, and speech is slurred. The patient may be feeling rage or apathy. Concentration, judgment, orientation, and memory are all impaired.

Physical assessment. It is essential that a physical examination be completed to rule out other medical complications such as head injury, cardiac dysrhythmia, bleeding, and pneumonitis.

Interventions

Provide a quiet environment and snack and coffee, which are helpful in calming the agitated patient.

Ensure that additional personnel are present before an assessment is attempted.

Attempt to establish disposition of the patient as quickly as possible.

Management of the violent patient is discussed later in this chapter.

Alcohol Withdrawal

Symptoms and signs of alcohol withdrawal range from mild discomfort (diaphoresis and tachycardia) to delirium that is life threatening. Delirium tremens resulting in death is caused by fluid deficiency, electrolyte imbalance, infection, and cardiac dysrhythmias. Withdrawal symptoms usually begin within 24 hours of the patient's last drink; therefore it is important to determine when the patient had the last drink. There is no consistent duration or severity of alcohol withdrawal.

Intervention

If it is established that the patient is in withdrawal from alcohol, the following medications should be promptly given: intramuscular thiamine 100 mg and chlordiazepoxide (Librium) 50 to 100 mg; if the patient remains uncomfortable or agitated, administer lorazepam 1 or 2 mg (by mouth or intramuscularly). Fluid and electrolyte imbalances must be corrected immediately.

THE VIOLENT PATIENT
The Patient at Risk

While all patients should be considered at risk for violence, there are those who represent a greater risk for assaultive behavior (Box 12–6). Because of the need for fairly intensive asstance, patients with organic brain disorder or dementia may strike out after an invasion of their personal space. A psychotic patient who is highly anxious may misinterpret the behavior of others. Alcohol or chemical substance abuse or intoxication places an individual at risk for violent behavior. Patients with personality disorders who have poor impulse control are capable of following through on verbal threats made to staff for not meeting their demands.

BOX 12–6	Warning Signs of Violent Behavior

VERBAL SIGNS

- Morose silence
- Short "yes" or "no" responses, not necessarily logical
- Negative responses to health care providers' requests
- Clipped and pressured speech
- Loudness
- Demanding, threatening language
- Giving a direct warning or threat
- Demeaning or derogatory statements

PHYSICAL SIGNS

- Facial expression: Jaws tense, teeth clenched, tightened lips; frowning; eyes vigilant, staring; flushed face; spitting
- Breathing: Shallow, rapid, irregular respirations
- Body language: Facing the health care provider; shaking, rocking back and forth; pacing; hitting or throwing objects; clenched fists; "stony" withdrawal; self-mutilation
- Affect and attitude: Sarcasm, paranoia, hostility, lability

Provocation

The issue of provocation may not be easily apparent but may

contribute to a patient's escalation of violent behavior and acting out. You can decrease the potential for violent, assaultive behavior by recognizing the following contributing factors to provocation and taking action to minimize or eliminate them:

> *Invasion of personal space.* People prone to violence require more personal space than others. Physically approaching a patient can look intrusive and increase the patient's anxiety or provoke aggression. Approaching a patient from behind may frighten the patient.
>
> *Failure to set limits.* Failure to set effective, *consistent* limits may lead to escalation of violent behavior and assault.
>
> *Negative or defensive staff attitude.* Attitudes such as aggressiveness and defensiveness and authoritarian behavior of staff toward patients can aggravate assaultive actions. Dislike and animosity, when projected toward a patient, can provoke the patient.

Assessment

Patients have individualized ways of expressing anger, frustration, and fear, and the cues that indicate potential or impending violent or assaultive behavior differ from patient to patient. Assess whether the patient's nonverbal behaviors are congruent with what the patient is saying.

Intervention

Three phases of intervention in response to a patient who is demonstrating violent behavior, progressing from the least to the most restrictive, are described in the following paragraphs.

Phase 1: Verbal deescalation. A staff member's ability to "talk the patient down" is enhanced by being able to communicate clearly and to interact in a confident, respectful manner. Using fundamental principles of assertive behavior and communication increases the likelihood of a successful outcome in potentially dangerous situations (Box 12–7). It is important to remain focused on what is occurring and what is needed by the patient. Refrain from moralistic or personal judgments, which

---

| BOX 12–7 | **Assertive Communication Skills** |

I. State what you have heard or observed
   A. Paraphrase what the patient has said.
   B. Describe what behaviors are being observed.

   Example: "I see that you are pacing and your face is
   flushed. I think it is beginning to frighten others around
   you. Can you tell me what is bothering you?"

II. Clearly state what you think, feel, and want from the patient.
   A. State limits and clarify expectations regarding new
      behaviors.
   B. Make clear, direct statements with specific information.
   C. Maintain eye contact.
   D. Use "I" statements.
   E. Be congruent in your behavior and message to the patient.

   Example: "I understand you are frustrated waiting an hour
   to see the physician, but do not yell and hit the desk. That
   behavior is not acceptable in the waiting room. I will go
   and see what the hold-up is and let you know. Go have a
   cigarette and I will be right back."

III. Avoid making statements such as the following: "You're
   freaking everybody out by acting so out of control. If you
   can't get your act together, I'll have you thrown out."

---

can contribute to the patient's increased anxiety and acting-out
behavior. Help the patient "problem-solve" the situation by
soliciting information regarding the patient's point of view, and
then validate the patient's concerns by paraphrasing what you
have heard. Suggest other helpful actions that may decrease the
patient's anger or anxiety, and observe how the patient responds
to you. If the patient's response indicates that the patient is
unable to maintain self-control, it may be necessary for staff to
progress to more restrictive forms of intervention in which con-
trols are externally imposed.

Phase 2: Chemical restraint. If verbal techniques prove fruitless, it is then appropriate to discuss the use of medications with the physician. These medications provide the patient with an antipsychotic, antianxiety, or sedative effect. In offering the psychotic patient medication, you will find the principles of assertiveness to be helpful. For the individual who is ''med-seeking,'' assessment and intervention are more difficult. These patients usually have a personality disorder and request the medication. Chemical restraint is *usually* more appropriate when the nonpsychotic individual does not ask for medication.

Patients always have the right to refuse medications unless they are committed to treatment by a court of law. Even in patients who are court committed, the types of medications a patient can be forced to take vary from state to state.

Phase 3: Physical restraint or "show of force." A psychiatric emergency exists when a patient is behaving in a way that presents a danger to self, others, or property. The ''show of force'' intervention is the most restrictive and is used only as a last resort when other interventions have failed. **However, a nurse *should not hesitate* to call for a show of force when a patient's violent behavior escalates too rapidly for the less restrictive approaches to be tried.** The show of force involves hospital staff physically removing the patient from the current location and restraining the patient with leather restraints that are either on a gurney or on a hospital bed. All hospitals should have a formal ''show of force'' policy and procedure (what intercom number to dial, what to say, who attends, and who leads the procedure), and the triage nurse should be very familiar with it.

It is often useful for the staff involved in a show of force to hold a debriefing session. Any personal injuries that may have occurred should be assessed. The leader or another designated person should ask the staff how effective they think the intervention was. Are any individuals emotionally upset? Is the staff ready to get back to work?

INVOLUNTARY TREATMENT

State laws vary from state to state about how persons are committed for psychiatric treatment against their will. Most states require that two physicians evaluate the patient and write a commitment order or that a police officer initiate the ''hold.'' Some states, like Washington, require that an independent mental health professional assess the patient. Reasons for involuntary hospital commitment, which do not vary, are listed in Box 12–8.

Any statements or observations relating to involuntary treatment should be documented promptly. Some states require that a written affidavit give the reason why a health care professional thinks a patient should be ''committed.'' In such states the nursing unit should provide an example of a completed affidavit and the procedure involved.

Nursing is a holistic profession that ''treats the patient, not just the disease.'' To some degree all nurses are ''med-psych'' nurses and should remain committed to feeling comfortable in performing all aspects of the patient's care. By practicing the

---

BOX 12–8 | **Reasons for Involuntary Hospitalization**

PATIENTS PRESENT A CLEAR AND PRESENT DANGER TO THEMSELVES

Suicidal patients with a strong desire to kill themselves and the means to do so if they left the hospital are often candidates. This type of commitment is uncommon in the ED. Depressed and suicidal patients who come to the hospital for an emergent admission are usually willing to be hospitalized. However, some do change their minds, commonly because of smoke-free psychiatric units.

PATIENTS PRESENT A CLEAR AND PRESENT DANGER TO OTHERS

Such patients range from the person with paranoia to an antisocial divorced man who is homicidal toward the man his former wife is dating. In the case of homicidal threats, threatened individuals should be notified. (This requirement varies from state to state.)

PATIENTS ARE "GRAVELY DISABLED"

Such patients are either grossly psychotic or have a debilitating brain disease such as Alzheimer's disease and are so confused or disorganized they are unable to care for their own basic needs.

MSE and being acutely aware of signs of escalating violence in patients' behavior, the triage nurse will be confident in assessing patients, and managing psychologic trauma, psychosis, suicidal ideation, overt hostility, intoxication, and panic, and, on a particularly challenging shift, providing care for someone who has all of the preceding disorders.

REFERENCE

American Psychiatric Association: *Diagnostic and statistical manual of mental disorders,* ed 4, Washington, DC, 1994, The Association.

RECOMMENDED READING

Blair DT: Assaultive behavior: does provocation begin in the front office? *J Psychosoc Nurs* 29(5):21, 1991.

Dubin W, Stolberg R: *Emergency psychiatry for the house officer,* New York, 1981, Spectrum.

Pokorny AD: Prediction of suicide in psychiatric patients, *Arch Gen Psychiatry* 40(2):279, 1983.

Rosenberg R, Kesselman M: The therapeutic alliance and the psychiatric emergency room, *Hosp Community Psychiatry* 44(1):78, 1993.

Slaby AE: *Handbook of psychiatric emergencies,* ed 4, Norwalk, Conn, 1994, Appleton & Lange.

Stevenson S: Heading off violence with verbal de-escalation. *J Psychosoc Nurs* 29(9):6, 1991.

13 | Triage: Ethics, Ideals, and Practice

Myriad opportunities exist for professional and personal enrichment and growth through the experience of triaging patients. Learning to make accurate decisions about patient acuity is an evolving process. Being able to triage well depends on assessment skills, a broad knowledge base, experience, and intuition. Individuals who triage must also have a willingness to learn from their mistakes, be compassionate and human, and reflect on the meaning of making decisions dealing with human life. As mentioned in Chapter 1, developing intuition takes time. The primary characteristic of the intuitive nurse is an open attitude toward people (Young [cited in Correnti, 1992]). Intuition develops as a nurse sees patterns of presentations and takes time to follow up on patients who have been triaged to learn about their diagnoses, treatments, and dispositions. Intuition may lead the nurse to make spontaneous conclusions, detect omitted data or gaps in data, or see relationships between pieces of information. Intuition may lead the nurse to make decisions based on the intuitive outcome rather than on what is strictly based in fact (Ruth-Sahd, 1993). Intuition also is fine tuned and shaped by the professional's ability to recognize and learn from her/his mistakes. Only in an ideal situation would all patients arrive at triage with classic patterns of illness or injury that are easy to assess, describe, and designate as the appropriate acuity level. Because patients are sometimes difficult to assess, have atypical patterns of presentation, or are evaluated on a day in which the triage professional is less than completely astute, triage decisions may be made that are less than helpful, occasionally harmful, and, rarely, downright dangerous to the patient's functioning or life. Unless professionals are willing to admit to themselves, to their colleagues, and to their patient, ''I made a mistake,'' they do not learn and grow as professionals, and they are not acting in an ethical and caring manner. Mistakes may be the result of poor judgment, inadequate knowledge, or inattention to detail, and they must be analyzed in attempts to keep from making the same mistake a second time (Kinney, 1992). The emergency department (ED) should be a supportive environment where individuals can discuss mistakes that are made in light of the specific situation and with consideration for staffing patterns, work load, job preparation, and other environmental factors in triage that may increase the risk of triage mistakes.

Ethical issues frequently arise in the practice of triage. Ethics is the science and art of determining the right and correct action to take in the context of the principles of professional practice and the good of the patient and the community. Ethics in triage requires an adaptation of a code that is founded on principles of equality, objectivity, and a concern that quality service is offered to each patient based on a truthful, fair, and expert appraisal of the patient's condition and need for services. The basics of ethical practice in American health care are summarized in Box 13–1.

Triage professionals often experience pressure to alter the way in which they assign triage acuity, which may challenge standards of ethical practice. These pressures include pressures regarding reimbursement based on verbiage necessary for services to be approved by insurance agencies, pressures from physicians and other health care colleagues who feel obligated to pursue unnecessary avenues of care precipitated by the triage professional's initial appraisal and documentation on a patient, pressures from patients who are emotionally distressed or who emphasize physical symptoms in order to influence the triage professional's triage acuity, and pressures from family members who may want to override a patient's wishes regarding the patient's health care. Legal standards often provide clear guidance for the triage nurse in coping with pressures at work that seek to influence triage care. George and Quattrone (1992) reviewed guidelines for patient's rights in ED care, as follows: "Patients who are conscious, oriented, and otherwise competent have the right to accept or refuse any treatment offered by emergency care providers . . . even if the emergency nurse feels the treatment is necessary to save the patient's life." Pressures must be dealt with on a case-by-case basis.

BOX 13–1	**The Basics of Ethical Practice in Health Care**

AUTONOMY

The ability for a competent individual to decide what will be done to his or her own body without coercion or threat

BENEFICENCE

Doing good or producing benefits for the patient in concordance with the patient's wishes

NONMALEFICENCE

Avoiding actions that are harmful to the patient

DISTRIBUTIVE JUSTICE

Comparable individuals sharing comparably in the benefits and burdens of the society

CONFIDENTIALITY

Information being held in confidence by members of the health care team unless there is a legal mandate to report patient information

PERSONAL INTEGRITY

Adherence to one's moral and professional standards

FIDELITY

The truth prevailing while cultural variables and patient's wishes are respected regarding assertive verbal communication of medical truths

Modified from Iserson K: *Emerg Med Clin North Am* 11(2):531, 1993.

Internal issues that influence the ethics of triage professionals include personal prejudices about ethnic groups or individuals with sexual orientation differing from what the professionals believe is acceptable, age-based prejudice, and political and economic concerns regarding the use, overuse, or underuse of emergency services. Although some triage professionals and individuals working in emergency services may deny the realty of ethical conflicts, observation of any health

---

| BOX 13–2 | **Tests for Judging the Ethical Viability of an Action or Triage Applications** |

IMPARTIALITY TEST

Would the practitioner have this action performed if in the patient's place? In triage, would the triage nurse have herself/ himself triaged in the manner and with the acuity designation that she/he determined for the patient?

UNIVERSALITY TEST

Would the practitioner feel comfortable having all practitioners perform this action in all relevant, similar circumstances? In triage, would the triage nurse feel comfortable with all triage nurses doing the triage assessment, interventions, and designation that she/he has performed on the patient?

INTERPERSONAL JUSTIFIABILITY TEST

Can the practitioner supply good reasons to others for his/her actions? In triage, can the triage nurse give good reasons for his/ her actions? Have the consequences and benefits for each option for the patient been considered and weighed?

Modified from Iserson K: *Emerg Med Clin North Am* 11(2):531, 1993.

---

care delivery facility in any 24-hour period would reveal that ethical conflicts are real. When they are not openly acknowledged and discussed, patient and community services suffer. Tests for judging whether triage decisions are ethical are listed in Box 13–2.

STANDARDS FOR EMERGENCY TRIAGE PRACTICE

Standards for emergency triage practice must include recognition of the following factors, which influence patient care in the triage setting.

1. Persons performing triage are enabled and limited in their professional practice by the terms of licensure and professional guidelines by which they practice, whether it be dictated by the board of registered nursing, board of licensed vocational or practical nursing, or paramedic or emergency

medical technician licensure. Professionals enacting triage are personally responsible for being familiar with the guidelines of professional practice by which they are licensed. Making medical diagnoses and implementing interventions beyond their scope of practice increase legal liability and are errors that are both illegal and unethical, since deception of the patient is inherently involved. While the professional may recognize that presenting signs and symptoms of illnesses or injuries are characteristics of a particular medical diagnosis, it is the responsibility of the triage professional to recognize the patient's acuity level, document and validate this appropriately, and triage the patient for appropriate care. Timely communication and documentation of same, with the ED physician when indicated, are crucial and reduce legal liability of the triage nurse (McLean, 1993).

2. The role of the professional responsible for triage is defined by the written job description for triage personnel of the agency. Each person performing triage must be familiar with the expectations defined for triage (including telephone triage) by the agency. Unless the person performing triage is also a unit manager, it is important that all decisions in triage requiring management verification or decision making be appropriately deferred and this delegation reflected in the patient's record. Likewise, the relationship between the triage professional and the physician supervising the medical care of patients should be clear so that consultation for triage decisions is available as needed and the triage professional knows how to access medical opinion when needed.

3. Triage professionals are bound by the policies and procedures of the agency and community in which they work. Policies directly written for triage are of primary relevance on a day-to-day basis, but procedures outlined by the facility's management and health care staff that are also relevant include care procedures for the treatment of common illnesses and injuries and outlined procedures for accessing primary health care providers and third-party payers regarding approval for patient services at the facility. Al-

though the latter may be the role of clerical staff in some facilities, it is helpful for the triage professional to be familiar with the process in the event that a patient who is denied permission for services by a third-party payer has an acuity level that is too high for safe triage out or transfer to another facility. It is the ethical and legal responsibility of the triage professional to advocate the appropriate level of care for the patient. If a patient is transferred from one facility to another with the primary impetus being fiscal concerns, a violation of the Consolidated Omnibus Budget Reconciliation Act (COBRA) may exist. COBRA is a provision of section 1867 of the Social Security Act, which was written to protect individuals from being "dumped" (Baier, 1993). Section 1867 is presented, in part, in Box 13–3.

Triage nurses, along with the ED staff and physicians, are responsible for being informed about and complying with COBRA. Because the law prohibits delay in screening to obtain financial information, triage should always be accomplished before financial information is sought from the patient (Baier, 1993). If patients are transferred, care must be taken to succinctly record the reason and time of the transfer, the condition

---

BOX 13–3	**Section 1867 of the COBRA Act**

In the case of a hospital that has a hospital emergency department, if any individual (whether or not eligible for benefits under this subchapter) comes to the emergency department and request is made on the individual's behalf for examination or treatment for a medical condition, the hospital must provide for an appropriate medical screening examination within the capability of the hospital's emergency department, including ancillary services routinely available to the emergency department, to determine whether or not an emergency medical condition (within the meaning of subsection [e] [1] of this section) exists.

From Section 1867 (42 U.S.C. 1395dd) (a).

of the patient, and communication with the patient and receiving facility. Communication with patients regarding the reason for an interfacility transfer or triage out of the facility must be done with care (Tammelleo, 1992c), and facilities may choose to inform patients that they may insist on ED care at the facility to which they have presented themselves.

There are times when patients "abuse the system." To achieve a specific purpose, some patients knowingly provide the triage nurse with an incomplete history or may omit information about their care that the primary health care provider may later share with the triage professional. Depending on the triage professional's access to primary health care information or old records, the triage nurse may need to reevaluate the patient in light of a more complete understanding of the patient's health problems, needs, and history. Ultimately the triage professional advocates what she/he believes is the most helpful and appropriate care for the patient.

The wishes of the patient, not those of the family or health care providers, are central to decisions regarding patient care. For example, if a patient has a valid advance directive or living will indicating her/his choice for resuscitative actions to be withheld or to be enacted, the patient's will supersedes the family's wishes (Adams et al., 1992). It is hoped that the two will not be in conflict. The triage nurse must always designate critically ill patients as emergent while communicating and providing a copy of living wills or advance directives, as available, on the patient's chart.

If a patient is denied access to emergency services (by an insurance representative or the patient's primary health care provider), the triage professional documents the actions taken to communicate the patient's status and perceived needs, names in the chart the professionals the triage professional has spoken with, and indicates the direction of patient triage requested by the consulting professional. If the triage professional works for a private hospital that is close to a public hospital and patients arriving for care in triage do not have the necessary insurance to receive services, the triage nurse is professionally obligated to ensure that the patient's condition is stable enough for the patient to receive care elsewhere. In all patients who have more than a nonurgent acuity level the presentations should be discussed with a physician, that is, the triage professional should consult with a physician in order to make the safest decision that services the patient's needs and is in agreement, whenever possible, with the facility's policies and procedures and in compliance with COBRA.

DIFFICULTIES IN TRIAGE

Difficulties in triage are frequently the result of the following scenarios.

1. The triage professional is inexperienced, is not fully oriented to her/his role in triage, and is unsure about how triage designation is determined.

An inexperienced or poorly informed triage nurse may see that there are various levels of acuity and figure out that "red" means that the patient is truly in need of emergent services but otherwise be unsure about how decisions are made based on the patient's history, presentation, and (in some situations) consultation with the patient's primary health care provider. If the triage professional has minimal assessment skills, he/she may triage patients based on their chief complaint and not on their overall presentation and risks based on their overall presentation in triage. When this occurs, a patient with a chief complaint of ankle swelling may be triaged to orthopedics as urgent when the true problem is congestive heart failure. A patient with a low-grade fever and shortness of breath may mistakenly be triaged to a clinic as nonurgent when she/he has a tubercular lesion and pneumothorax.

It is the responsibility of management to ensure that professionals who will be triaging patients have a clear understanding of assessment, a sound knowledge base in illness and injury, and an understanding of triage policies and procedures. Furthermore, the triage nurse should be encouraged to consult with a physician or nurse-manager when a patient is difficult to triage or an accurate acuity level is difficult to assign. Conversely, the ED manager should respect and foster intuitive decisions made by the triage nurse regarding patient acuity. The ED manager should particularly offer guidance to the inexperienced triage nurse and give supportive guidance in verifying or changing triage designations that fit the patient. As Benner

(1984) has identified in her book *From Novice to Expert,* the beginning practitioner often has difficulty in prioritizing patient care. Therefore it is again recommended that only experienced nurses be oriented and perform in the role of triage nurse (Ruth-Sadh, 1993). The beginning nurse can be taught to follow protocols, but since intuitive judgment is a critical aspect of triage care, this skill should be fostered through affirmation of the nurse who makes intuitive judgments in the triage area. An ED atmosphere that is conducive to discussion and questioning is a positive arena for development of intuitive sense.

2. The triage professional is tired or ''burned out'' and therefore ineffective and unsympathetic.

The preceding scenario is dangerous, not only to the effective implementation of triage but also to the reputation of the facility that employs the professional in triage. When triage nurses are not functioning optimally, communication that is not helpful or is even rude can take place during stressful situations. In one lawsuit, in which the plaintiff won $450,000, the plaintiff was told in the ED that ''if he did not like the way the hospital was being run, he should go to another hospital'' (Tammelleo, 1992b). Since the patient was not informed of the potential hazards of leaving without care, a breach in standards of care was found. It is helpful for management to consider the number of hours for which a nurse is asked to triage, particularly in busy EDs with long waiting periods for patients. Patients in the waiting area often feel that the triage professional is personally responsible for their prolonged suffering, and some angrily denounce the triage person as uncaring or as power-mongering (typically using other, less kind terms). It is helpful for one nurse to triage for several hours, to provide continuity of care for patients who need periodic reevaluation and retriage according to changes in their condition. Triage nurses have been exculpated in cases in which emergent patients have had to wait for prompt ED care, when clear documentation of appropriate triage designation was evident and the times when the patient's situation had been communicated with the ED manager were documented (Tammelleo, 1992a). Patient reevaluation in the waiting room is best performed by the individual who originally triaged the patient. However, a clear report made by the professional who is leaving a triage shift to assume another role within the ED to an oncoming triage nurse permits continuity of care in any units where nurses change shifts. Four-hour triage duty is sufficient in many EDs, and 6-hour duty is the maximum acceptable number of hours in a busy ED. Eight or 12 hours in triage is a reasonable shift in EDs or facilities where strain or stress caused by these prolonged shifts has not been identified as a problem by staff performing triage. Management appraisal of the number of hours for which staff should triage should be based on staff feedback, direct observation of triage professionals and patients in the triage area, and patient feedback. ED management also must periodically review conditions that precipitate ''burnout,'' in particular commitment to career, collegial relations, and job satisfaction (Stechmiller and Yarandi, 1993). Opportunities for career growth have a trickle-down effect on triage excellence. Collegial relations should be positive and modeled by positive management skills, and feedback and factors influencing job satisfaction should be defined through discussions with staff, with changes to the triage environment, policies, and procedures implemented when appropriate.

3. The professional designated to perform triage is not comfortable with the role.

Some professionals are not well suited to triage because they have difficulty sorting individuals with a variety of complaints and are confused by the constant interruptions that may occur in a busy triage area, such as interruptions by family members of other patients being cared for in the ED, telephone calls, and patients who are anxious for services and want to know when they will be seen. Some individuals are linear thinkers who cannot cope with the frenetic environment in a busy triage area, and they should have the opportunity to request that they not be required to perform triage.

4. Resources in the facility are inadequate.

Triage may be inaccurate, difficult, and downright dangerous to the professional's liability and personal comfort and safety if the facility does not recognize and meet the needs involved in creating an effective triage environment. Triage professionals should have safe conditions in which to practice at all times. This means that security should be readily accessible should a patient or others become violent or threatening toward the triage nurse, one another, or anyone in the waiting area. Triage professionals should also have a ready exit route in case they must flee for their own safety. And in EDs where violence has consistently been a problem, police protection should be available at all times. Triage professionals should not have to fight for these rights—it is the ethical responsibility of the agency to ensure a safe environment at all times for its employees and consumers.

In facilities with a high number of non–English-speaking patients, translators should be available whenever possible or the method for accessing a translator by telephone should be clearly posted. If triage professionals are unable to communicate with patients who arrive for care, it may be impossible or at best difficult to accurately determine the patients' chief complaints, not to mention information regarding allergies and other critical information. When there is a high number of patients with a specific second language, consideration should be given to hiring a translator to permit triage and care to be safely conducted.

5. Patients may seek services under false pretenses or may be unreliable historians.

It is impossible to be precisely accurate in determining the necessary level of care for patients who lie about their histories or fake physical symptoms to access care. While it is not the responsibility of the triage professional to figure out whether a patient is lying, it is important that indicators of unreliability be documented on the triage record. Although certain behaviors may indicate unreliability to the triage professional (e.g., a patient is unable to maintain eye contact), consideration to various ethnic backgrounds and individual norms must be given, and any indicator that may be construed as subjective should not be recorded on the triage record. Only indicators that can be objectively recorded should become part of the permanent record. For example, when a patient arrives at the ED with a chief complaint of chest pain and is immediately seen in triage but then denies chest pain and complains of stomach cramps, both complaints should be recorded in the patient's own words. Since the patient immediately denied the initial chief complaint on arrival in triage, this should be recorded also. The reason for recording this information is not to make the patient "look bad" but to indicate that the patient has a complicated presentation and to forewarn care providers that diagnosis and treatment may be particularly challenging in the patient. It is not the responsibility of the triage professional to look beyond the patient's behavior and figure out the reasons for unreliability, but it is important to remember that there are many reasons for this problem. The patient should not be judged but rather should be treated with kindness and objectivity.

Some patients are unreliable historians because they are afraid. They may be afraid of what will be done to obtain a diagnosis or treat them. If they are injured or ill as a result of neglect or battery by a family member or significant other, they may be afraid—for themselves or their children—that negative consequences may be waiting at home if the perpetrator is implicated for maltreatment of the patient. Some patients are unreliable simply because they have poor memories or are mentally confused. Still others are seeking drugs and arrive with complaints that are tailor-made to achieve the purpose of receiving narcotics. If the triage nurse suspects that a patient's delay in care has been intentional and has resulted in the illness becoming highly acute, this concern must be communicated with the ED manager and supervising ED physician. In the case of children or individuals who are under conservatorship, criminal charges may be filed if there has been "failure to exercise due care in the treatment of another, where a duty to furnish such care exists" (Fiesta, 1992b). It is a legal and an ethical responsibility to act as an advocate for the child or patient under conservatorship. If the triage nurse feels that the home care provider is at risk for leaving with the patient from the waiting area before being seen in the ED, designation of a higher triage acuity level may be necessary for the ultimate safety of the patient, and the patient should be transferred into the ED without delay.

The manner in which patients who repeatedly seek narcotics through emergency services are identified in the emergency health care system varies from state to state and from facility to facility. Some facilities keep a log of "system abusers" so that they can be triaged back to their primary care providers if they seek services for pain medication. Other facilities do not keep a record but contact the patient or primary health care provider or both to request that the patient not seek treatment for pain at the ED. This issue is sensitive and rightly so because health care providers in emergency services do not want to deny access to care in the event of a "real" medical illness or injury but neither do they want to reinforce the patient's addiction by rewarding him/her with attention and treatment for a self-induced or false presentation initiated with the intent of receiving narcotics. Patients with addictions are best served by recognition of their problem and triage of the patients back to a primary care provider, who will remind the patients of the availability of addiction treatment options and pain clinics or treatment centers if the patient truly has some form of chronic or recurring pain. The best way to identify and treat individuals who overuse emergency services is to perform routine chart audits for identified chief complaints or to attend to the identification by staff of an individual who is consistently using emergency services for primary health care. The reason for the behavior can then be identified with the patient by an administrator and the primary health care provider, and alternatives for more appropriate, continuous health care and monitoring can be offered.

PREVENTION

Prevention is the key to avoiding mistakes and unethical decision-making practices in the triage area. The "utopia of triage" would have characteristics like those that follow.

1. The triage area is clean, well lit, and stocked with all the necessary equipment.

For thorough triage decision making the following are all available and in immediate proximity to the triage area: a scale, thermometers, blood pressure cuff, pulse oximeter, one-touch glucose-level monitoring device, urine dip stick, rapid urine pregnancy testing kit, and bathroom. The following first aid and comfort equipment is also neatly stored in triage drawers or cupboards readily accessible to the professional: tissues, basins for emesis (large, not the half-cup size), bandages, Ace wraps, gloves, protective blue pads, linens, and acetaminophen. Wheel chairs are just outside the triage area, and a gurney is ready at all times. An emergency obstetric delivery kit is available for deliveries in the parking lot or triage area that cannot be avoided by even the deftest of triage professionals. A telephone with several lines is available. A copy of the triage policies is on hand. Essential triage information tools are handy (estimated-date-of-confinement wheel, growth and development information, acetaminophen-dosing chart, vital sign norms for pediatric patients by age, and so forth). A list of telephone numbers for contacting primary health care providers and insurance personnel is in triage. A hotline to the police department and security is within easy reach. A computer is in the triage area. A cot and diapers are available for small infants.

2. The triage area is staffed by an experienced registered nurse or nurse practitioner and a bilingual aide who is qualified as a translator and medical assistant or nurse's aide. Security is readily available or near the triage area at all times to ensure the safety of triage personnel.
3. The triage area is directly accessible to the care area, and patients designated as emergent can easily be brought into the care area without a physical challenge to the triage staff.
4. The ED or supervising physician is available for consultation.
5. Clerical staff who must assist the triage professional are physically near the triage professional for communication and added assistance as needed.
6. Triage policies, procedures, and reference manuals are available in the triage area.
7. Separate waiting cubicles are available for patients who require isolation because of the potential for contagion.
8. The waiting area is clean, well lit, and quiet.
9. Work breaks are ensured and are provided for triage personnel by ED managers.
10. Follow-up calls are possible, as is follow-up on patients from whom the triage professionals may learn about treatments, outcomes, and the appropriateness of triage designations.

When the physical environment is optimal and the triage nurse knows his/her responsibilities, governing policies and procedures, and resources, the job of triaging is made easier.

An atmosphere within the ED that is conducive to ethical practice is also necessary if triage is to be conducted in an honest, ethical, and helpful manner.

In the health care setting it is essential that patients and health care providers have a basic trust of one another. If agencies agree that honesty is the best policy, it is important to avoid entrapping triage professionals into telling lies or perverting the truth by manipulating, however slightly, triage data to serve the best interest of patient or the agency. Policies regarding triage practice should not conflict with the safety and good of patients. All regulations (policies and procedures) must be consistent with principles that recognize an individual's right to seek treatment and be treated with dignity. This is not to say that it is neither helpful nor appropriate to have policies and procedures for triaging patients "out" to more appropriate health care agencies, but that the patient's best interests are at the forefront of policy making. In the United States today there are limited legislated rights to health care for some individuals with certain diagnoses, but no patient can legally claim a right to "universal" health care (Knopp et al., 1992).

Since as many as 36 million Americans do not have health insurance and many more are underinsured, ED personnel are under a great deal of pressure and are ethically obligated to serve, even if in a limited way, the needs of the medically indigent.

Enacting policies and procedures in triage depends on cooperation and mutual respect among triage professionals, physicians, administrators, and insurance agencies. Manipulation of triage language (e.g., the patient's chief complaint or description of the patient's symptoms) should not be necessary to achieve the appropriate level of care a patient honestly needs. Although direct health care providers, triage professionals, patients, and business persons may see a health care problem from a variety of perspectives, all should be willing to be open to one another's concerns and limitations. Each individual must answer to the licensing requirements and laws that govern practice in the state in which she/he resides. Any triage nurse who suspects that a patient will suffer deleterious consequences if denied services in the ED or who sees a patient who has possibly suffered consequences of intentional poor care or negligence has a legal duty to report this problem to his/her supervisor and document it in an "incident report" or another type of document used in the facility (Fiesta, 1992a).

If insurance agency personnel who are responsible for approving funding for emergency care are not qualified health care providers, they must trust the judgment of the triage professional who has performed a "live" appraisal of the patient. However, triage professionals must also be open to hearing the concerns of insurance personnel and patients before forming a response. In any event, discussions with insurance personnel or any health care personnel regarding a patient in triage should always be documented on the patient's record, including the name of the person with whom the triage nurse has consulted.

Triage professionals must be aware of personal prejudices that may cause them to be less than honest. These prejudices may be based on personal feelings, beliefs, or fears or on a need to feel accepted. For example, giving unrealistic estimates of waiting periods for those in the ED waiting area or telling a patient "you're next" when she/he may not be is not only dishonest but ultimately unkind, and such statements may not have the intended effect of assuring patients that they will soon receive care. A handout orienting patients to the ED, which includes possible impediments to their immediate treatment (e.g., patients arriving by ambulance, and critically ill patients), is helpful in reducing the responsibility a triage nurse may feel regarding prolonged waiting periods. Answering patients' questions regarding what the triage nurse thinks is wrong with them or what might happen to them is another aspect of triage care in which telling partial truths or assuming too much responsibility can be a pitfall of triage practice. If policies are clear regarding triage and treatment of a patient with a specific presentation, the triage nurse may tell the patient what area of the ED is most likely to be performing the evaluation, and patients may be told that they will be involved in decision making regarding diagnostic procedures and ultimately treatment of their condition.

Success of the triage professional in any health care setting depends on an ability to think clearly in a frenetic situation, an impressive knowledge base, excellent assessment skills, and the ability to designate triage acuity levels accurately. Success of the triage professional also depends on the professional's ability to impart compassion, treat patients and family members with kindness, respect each individual's right to dignity, and perform in an ethical, professional manner. Successful professionals deserve recognition from themselves, their colleagues, and their community for their valuable contribution. They perform a critical role in emergency services and are assets to the human race.

REFERENCES

Adams J et al: Ethical aspects of resuscitation, *Ann Emerg Med* 21(10):1273, 1992.

Baier FE: Implications of the Consolidated Omnibus Budget Reconciliation "antidumping" legislation for emergency nurses, *J Emerg Nurs* 19(2):115, 1993.

Benner PE: *From novice to expert: excellence and power in clinical nursing practice,* Reading, Mass, 1984, Addison-Wesley.

Correnti D: Intuition and nursing practice implications for nurse educators: a review of the literature, *J Contin Educ Nurs* 23(2):91, 1992.

Fiesta J: Criminal liability for the nurse. Part I. *Nurse Manage* 23(4):16, 1992a.

Fiesta, J, Criminal liability for the nurse. Part II. *Nurse Manage* 23(5):16, 1992b.

George J, Quattrone M: Restraining patients: can you be sued? Part I, *J Emerg Nurs* 18(6):536, 1992.

Iserson K: Ethical dilemmas in hematologic/oncologic emergencies, *Emerg Med Clin North Am* 11(2):531, 1993.

Kinney M: Error and mistake: inward gain or personal loss, *Focus Crit Care* 19(1):7, 9, 1992.

Knopp RK et al: An ethical foundation for health care: an emergency medicine perspective, *Ann Emerg Med* 21:1381, 1992.

McClean P: Lawsuits and nurses, *Can Nurse* 89(11):53, 1993.

Ruth-Sahd L: A modification of Benner's hierarchy of clinical practice: the development of clinical intuition in the novice trauma nurse, *Holist Nurs Pract* 7(3):8, 1993.

Stechmiller J, Yarandi H: Predictors of burnout in critical care nurses, *Heart Lung* 22(6):534, 1993.

Tammelleo A: $6.2 million verdict reversed: vicarious liability, *Regan Rep Nurs Law* 32(8):1, 1992a.

Tammelleo A: Patient misdiagnosed and invited to ''leave'': $450,000 verdict. Case in point: Baptist Memorial Hospital v. Bowen (591 So. 2d 74—AL [1991]), *Regan Rep Nurs Law* 32(10):4, 1992b.

Tammelleo A: How the law protects emergency patients, *RN* 55(10):67, 71, 1992c.

RECOMMENDED READING

Aiken TD, Catalano JT: *Legal, ethical, and political issues in nursing,* Philadelphia, 1994, Cavis.

Emergency Cardiac Care Committee and Subcommittees, American Heart Association: Guidelines for cardiopulmonary resuscitation and emergency cardiac care. Part VIII. Ethical considerations in resuscitation, *JAMA* 268(16):2282, 1992.

Hansten RI, Washburn M: *Clinical delegation skills,* Gaithersburg, Md, 1994, Aspen.

Renz M: Learning from intuition, *Nursing* 23(7):44, 1993.

Index